THE Sᴇχuᴀʟ P
ᴏꜰ Quᴏᴅᴄ

GW00507365

"Amara has a very special gift of being able to articulate these unique and insightful teachings that give real direction on how to heal and move forward as a sexual, spiritual being. She skillfully marries the disciplines of many cultures so that all may relate in some way and, therefore, receive benefit. This book is for anybody looking for expansion, expression, and a new path to enhance sex and intimacy in their lives."

LAURA KIMBRO, OB/GYN DO,
FELLOW OF THE AMERICAN COLLEGE OF OBSTETRICS

"Quodoushka's Fire Breath full-body orgasm was absolutely the most valuable thing I ever learned about sex. This hotly anticipated brave book is a treasure trove of wisdom that raises the bar on sex education. Amara Charles knows these practices intimately, and her enthusiasm for her subjects rubs off. Great for beginners to advanced."

ANNIE SPRINKLE, PH.D., AUTHOR OF
DR. SPRINKLE'S SPECTACULAR SEX

"Imagine if we grew up in a culture where we were taught about sexuality and learned to be great lovers and healthy human beings. In *The Sexual Practices of Quodoushka*, Amara Charles shares once secret teachings and information in a fun and entertaining way that will help save relationships, lives, and our planet. Read this book and give thanks!"

BABA DEZ NICHOLS, FOUNDER OF THE INTERNATIONAL SCHOOL
OF TEMPLE ARTS, AUTHOR OF *SACRED SEXUAL HEALING:*
THE SHAMAN METHOD OF SEX MAGIC

"*The Sexual Practices of Quodoushka* is a comprehensive introduction to a powerful way of connecting to and activating our inherent sexual potencies and abilities to experience pleasure. Amara Charles masterfully guides the reader through the cultural background of the practices into the realm of their concrete application, outlining a new understanding of sexual conditioning and experience while encouraging innovative ways of bringing greater pleasure into our lives. A thorough delight."

LIVIA KOHN, AUTHOR AND PROFESSOR EMERITA OF RELIGION
AND EAST ASIAN STUDIES AT BOSTON UNIVERSITY

"*The Sexual Practices of Quodoushka* beautifully complements the ancient knowledge of the Taoist shaman. These transformational teachings reveal ways to deepen and strengthen relationships and offer a means to access the universal healing forces of creation."

MASTER MANTAK CHIA, AUTHOR OF
HEALING LOVE THROUGH THE TAO AND *TAOIST FOREPLAY*

"With *The Sexual Practices of Quodoushka,* Amara Charles is helping to make our world a more peaceful and loving place. You will learn the Quodoushka teachings, which state that the lack of healthy sexual expression is the root cause of abusive, addictive, and violent behaviors. And you will learn specific steps you can take to transform your sex life into the sacred and healing practice it was meant to be!"

VERONICA MONET, ACS, CAM, CERTIFIED SEXOLOGIST, COUPLES
CONSULTANT, AND RADIO HOST OF *THE SHAME FREE ZONE*

"In *The Sexual Practices of Quodoushka*, Amara Charles captures the essence of intimacy. From personal experience I can say unequivocally that she is brilliant, knowledgeable, and an absolute cauldron of vital energy. This book will guide you to become a more caring lover, free blocked energy, and delight in your body to align your human, animal, and spiritual aspects. Charles's explanation of sexual anatomy types is a genuine revelation. *Sexual Practices of Quodoushka* can make a quantum shift in the way you approach sex and intimacy."

STEVEN BARNES, AUTHOR, LECTURER, AND MARTIAL ARTIST

"Quodoushka weekends led by Amara are always filled with indescribable sexual magick. With this book she combines a vivid literary style with her practical experience of working energetically through blocks to sexual enrichment. The wisdom rooted in the teachings of the elders comes alive on these pages. Amara has somehow captured their spiritual electricity."

RICHARD BECK PEACOCK, FILM DIRECTOR AND COAUTHOR OF
LEARNING TO LEAVE: A WOMAN'S GUIDE

"*The Sexual Practices of Quodoushka* is a tremendous resource for anyone trying to understand their own sexuality so that they can bring that sexuality to a relationship and participate fully in that relationship. How wonderful would it be if we could teach children sex through this voice as opposed to through television, the Internet, or pornography. I am of the belief that this would lead to far healthier sexual relationships as adults."

ALLEN N. CHIURA, M.D., UROLOGIST

THE
SEXUAL PRACTICES
·OF
QUODOUSHKA

Teachings from the Nagual Tradition

Amara Charles

Destiny Books
Rochester, Vermont • Toronto, Canada

Destiny Books
One Park Street
Rochester, Vermont 05767
www.DestinyBooks.com

Destiny Books is a division of Inner Traditions International

Library of Congress Cataloging-in-Publication Data
Charles, Amara.
  The sexual practices of Quodoushka : teachings from the Nagual tradition / Amara Charles.
     p. cm.
  Includes bibliographical references and index.
  Summary: "Practical exercises to reach higher levels of orgasm, renew relationships, and discover the healing power of sex"—Provided by publisher.
  ISBN 978-1-59477-357-0 (pbk.) — ISBN 978-1-59477-934-3
  1. Indians of Mexico—Sexual behavior. 2. Sex instruction. 3. Nagualism. I. Title.
  F1219.3.S45C47 2011
  972'.00497—dc23

                                                          2011021325

Printed and bound in the United States by Versa Press, Inc.

10   9   8   7   6

Text design and layout by Virginia Scott Bowman
This book was typeset in Garamond Premier Pro and Gill Sans with Mason Alternate and Gill Sans as display typefaces

To send correspondence to the author of this book, mail a first-class letter to the author c/o Inner Traditions • Bear & Company, One Park Street, Rochester, VT 05767, and we will forward the communication.

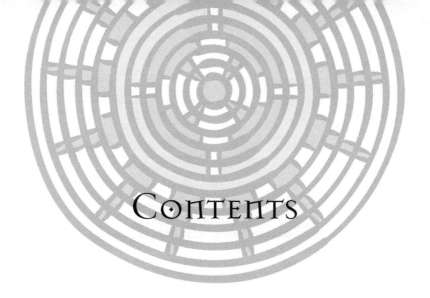

Contents

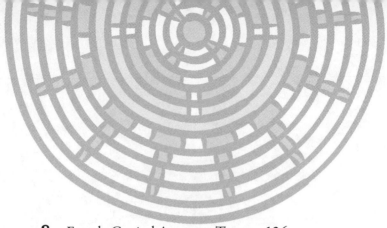

The spirit that created you is alive in you and is always present in all forms of all things.

FOREWORD

So many marriages and relationships fall apart because they lack a deep level of satisfaction, endearment, and endurance. Until we can learn how to use our sexual soul force energy as a catalyst to increase our sensitivity and connection to life, disappointment and disillusion will continue to destroy countless relationships. What's needed is a more tolerant environment where people of all sexual persuasions feel free to explore their inherent sexuality.

It is our challenge and our responsibility in this lifetime to transcend limitations of the past, for it is only through ignorance that we surrender our freedom. This is why it is so important to have a more empowered sexual education—not only through Quodoushka—but through other teachings that encompass the spiritual aspects of our sexuality as well.

Repression is hazardous to humanity, because when you repress a person's sexuality, you retard the maturation of their soul. Religions and political structures that restrict people from discovering their full potential as men and women thwart the evolution of humanity and make it impossible for people to discover who they really are. If you cannot fully express yourself and stand accountable for your actions, you cannot find the fulfillment that every human being deserves.

This book, which Amara has so beautifully written, goes a long way toward helping people lift themselves from the unknown and often unexamined territories of sexual knowledge and pleasure. The teachings and practices presented here are from the first two of the five levels of

Quodoushka workshops now available to the public. These Quodoushka teachings are designed to help people embrace their sexuality as a positive catalyst for change in their lives.

When you are able to experience high levels of orgasmic pleasure, you feel content with your place in the universe. You become more creative, more awake, aware, and alert. You have the energy to make things happen and your whole world changes into a better way of living.

How many men and women could benefit from learning that they don't have to go through relationships unconsciously or lose connection to their sexuality as they age? Quodoushka shows us that we can do something to sustain and increase our vitality in life. In order to remain healthy, full of energy, and to thrive in a world faced with perilous decisions that affect the freedoms of us all, we must be as close to God as we can be. Creation has designed the art of making love to be the fastest and most beautiful way for human beings to be able to touch spirit. Therefore, examine these teachings closely, question them with boldness, search for the truth, and find your own way into the heart of your circle of self.

THUNDER STRIKES,
TWISTED HAIRS NAQUAL ELDER

Acknowledgments

I sincerely thank Thunder Strikes and Dianne Nightbird for their generous support and unbending intent to preserve and bring forth the knowledge contained in this book, and for all they have done to ensure that it continues to evolve for future generations. Thunder Strikes is responsible for articulating the entire body of Quodoushka teachings in its modern form. Without the courage, guidance, and vision of both of these individuals, this book would not have been possible.

I thank my fellow Quodoushka teachers and the support teams whose years of dedication have helped many people experience the beauty of these practices. My boundless gratitude goes to Shyena Venice for standing by my side while I wrote this book. Special thanks go to Sheryl McIntyre, Jeffrey Fine, Steven Barnes, George Basch, Richard Peacock, David Capco, Tom McGrew, Jan Holmes, Janneke Koole, Sharman Okan, Carol Briskin, Susan Oake, Belinda Duffy, Marguerite Mullins, Leela Sullivan, Mukee Okan, and Sherry Folb, all of whom played special parts in helping this book come to be.

I bow in sincere gratitude to the many Quodoushka graduates who have kept these teachings alive by sharing them with their families and friends. While I have chosen to change the names of various contributors for privacy's sake, I have done my best to keep the essence of their stories intact. Finally, many thanks to those who helped me gain an intimate knowledge of the sexual anatomy types.

Introduction

THE MEDICINE OF SEX

Learning Through Pleasure

It is said that when a teaching "grows corn" it has value and makes your life better; otherwise it is useless. So much of what we have been taught about sex does not grow corn in our relationships, and too often it leaves us disappointed, frustrated, and unfulfilled. What's needed is a clear understanding of how to use the powerful yet delicate energy of sex.

Thinking we already know all there is to know about sex is the biggest obstacle to enjoying greater intimacy. Typically, it occurs to us that we have a lot to learn only after a relationship crashes or when nothing we try seems to work. Even though we may wish to have more fulfilling sexual experiences, where do we go for practical guidance? What does it take to successfully balance our intimate desires along with everything else going on in our lives? Where do we turn if our sexual feelings are locked inside yearning to be expressed?

Since most of us come from families where meaningful guidance was scant if it existed at all, many are hungry to find sensible approaches for creating healthy sexual relationships. For me, discovering the teachings and practices of Quodoushka dramatically changed the course of my life. They not only offered an inspiring system of integrated knowledge, they expanded my whole view of sex, orgasms, and relationships. They helped me accept the unique characteristics of my sexual anatomy and, most importantly, showed me how we can

1

learn through pleasure to become more sensitive, creative lovers.

Since 1978 Quodoushka, in its modern form, has followed the custom of ancient traditions in which information was spread mostly by word of mouth. Thus, over twenty years ago, when a friend told me about this workshop, I called to find out what it was. I believe I may hold the world's record for being cajoled to attend. I rambled on about my uncertainties and offered every possible reason why it was impossible for me to attend, but after listening to my own resistance for several hours, it was obvious what was really so. I was pretty confused and I needed some answers, but I was terrified to face my sexuality.

I calmed down considerably on the first night when I heard the facilitator, Elizabeth Chandra, a doctor from California, say in her introduction, "I advise you to not believe anything I am going to tell you. If you do, you are a fool. No," she said, "please do not believe. Question everything. When something is true for you, you will feel it. Truth is not merely seen or heard, it must be felt by you."

Thunder Strikes, the founder of the Quodoushka teachings, says, "Your sex is natural. It's for your health." And then he explains, "Great Spirit gives human beings two sacred gifts that make us different from the animal world. One is the gift of free will, and we are free to do as we will. The other is the gift of orgasm. Animals have sex to reproduce; they don't create romantic evenings to have orgasms. The human body however, is *designed* to feel pleasure. Why did Great Spirit make our orgasms so pleasurable, and why do so many people feel guilty or shameful about sex? Orgasms are given to us for two reasons; they allow us to feel pleasure and help us gain knowledge of who we truly are."

This, along with many other Quodoushka teachings, was a far cry from what I was told growing up as a girl in the Midwest suburbs. Up to that point, no one in my life had ever mentioned that sex could be something spiritual or transcendent. Like so many others to whom I have presented these teachings, sex was something I managed well enough, but more often than not, it became a source of difficulty and suffering.

It is the ring of truth I felt from these words that shaped my life toward understanding and embodying a spiritually sexual life, that is, a life that feels connected with nature and that treats sex as something healthy and good. It is also what led me to become an apprentice and a teacher within this tradition many years ago.

THE SHAMANIC APPROACH OF CHULUAQUI QUODOUSHKA

The shamanic approach provides hands-on, experiential practices that peel away the contrivances of social conditioning and cut through our habitual perceptions. *Chuluaqui Quodoushka,* the full name of these teachings, brings us back in touch with the natural sexual feelings we have lost touch with. The word *Chuluaqui* (pronounced Choo-la-kway) refers to the primordial life-force energy that comprises and courses through everything. *Quodoushka* (pronounced kwuh-DOE-shka) means the union of two energies coming together to generate more than the sum of individual parts. Quodoushka teaches that sexual energy is the most powerful way to directly feel the original energy from which each of us is born. Far more than a set of dry instructions, Quodoushka shows us how to appreciate our sexual energy as sacred and profound. It offers a way to heal sexual wounds, and it is a path of learning how to sustain endearing relationships.

One of the things that makes Quodoushka's approach to sexuality unique, and perhaps a reason it has flourished worldwide for so many years, is the inherent understanding that for each of us to feel connected to our source we must be willing to face our shadows. Hidden in the unseen corners of self, where we suppress pleasure and hold back the fullness of our sexual feelings, are memories of accumulated guilt, blame, and shame. Like our shadows and wounds, for corn to grow, it's first buried in the dark earth. Then it must be nourished with the light of understanding and tended with creative actions. Quodoushka is a compassionate way to learn about sex, and it has been called the path of the wounded healer.

Herein lies the mystery of sex, for whether it is reined into a dark corner of our lives, reveled in, or neglected, it is an undeniably powerful force. When we exploit its power, or avoid its natural expression for too long, it turns into a poison. According to Quodoushka, excessive repression is the major reason for disharmony in relationships; and furthermore, the lack of healthy sexual expression is the root cause of abusive, addictive, and violent behaviors. Because it is clear that misuse of sexual energy harms the human body, spirit, and mind, Quodoushka emphasizes the need to approach sex with responsibility and wisdom. It is only when we take responsibility for our sexuality that we can learn to use it as a healing medicine.

NOT WITHOUT CONTROVERSY

The presentation of these practices by Quodoushka's pioneer, Thunder Strikes, and the team of instructors he and Dianne Nightbird have authorized to present Quodoushka throughout the United States, Canada, Europe, and the Asian Pacific, has not been without controversy. Critical comments have been made by those who object to non–Native American men and women sharing sexuality teachings that are said to be derived from ancient Cherokee and Navaho practices as well as Mayan, Toltec, and other pre-Christian sources.

Wikipedia currently posts a statement by Dr. Richard Allen, a research and policy analyst of the Cherokee Nation, which implies, of Quodoushka, that Thunder Strikes made it up. He goes on to say, "We learn about sex like everyone else does, behind the barn."[1] There are critics who deny that any ancient sexuality teachings come from Native American tribes, and they reject the notion that their ancestors created an intricate body of knowledge supported by the vast collection of remarkably precise observations regarding human sexuality that are revealed in forthcoming chapters of this book.

Part of the difficulty in tracing these teachings' distinct place of origin lies in the fact that they were passed from teacher to student throughout many generations, and there are, to my knowledge, no written documents currently available to substantiate their claims. Thunder Strikes is the first to acknowledge that Quodoushka teachings do not come from one tribe, or one individual; rather, they are collected from those who are called Twisted Hairs Elders. He refrains from claiming sole authorship and views himself more as a spokesman for his teachers, the Twisted Hairs Nagual* Elders of the Sweet Medicine Sundance Path of Turtle Island, who he says prefer to remain anonymous.

Yet the clues remain. One has only to look at the records retained in the iconography and art relics of ancient Mayan and Toltec civilizations for testimony that sexuality was a vital aspect of their lives. Sculptures such as the large stelae of Mesoamerica showing phalluses and female figures with enlarged breasts and genitals suggest the significance of fertility, and hence the importance of sexuality, dating back thousands of years. The heritage of Quodoushka stems from these pre-Christian cultures, in which sexuality was likely as necessary to understand as it is in today's world.

Westerners must frequently turn to the East, to Asian sources, and to ancient models from indigenous people to find a more holistic, positive, and practical approach to sex. Whether it's due to issues of morality, religion, or social values, our culture has avoided developing meaningful sexual education beyond what's necessary for procreation. Even so, as evidenced by the recent surge of seniors wanting to enjoy sex well into their later years, and the interest in Tantra by people of all ages, many are seeking to learn alternative ways to have more satisfying sexual lives.

Bringing the sense of a "spiritual" quality to sex is perhaps a new idea to some. By spiritual we do not mean religious in any sense of the word. Spiritual sexuality means—and Quodoushka teaches—to be responsible, kind, and respectful in our sexual relationships. We leave up to the reader to decide whether pinpointing their exact place of origin is relevant to their effectiveness. Listen for the ring of truth, explore new things about yourself, and see what grows corn in your life.

---

*Nagual (pronounced Nah-Whal) is a warrior-magician-shaman who has the ability to change his or her appearance. In Mesoamerican folk tales this has been depicted as a person with the ability to shapeshift into a crow, a turtle, or even a dragon. However, Quodoushka uses the term to describe a healer and sage of the highest order; someone who can transform from one state to another, heal sicknesses, and who ultimately strives to reach the highest states of humanity not by turning into an animal, but by transforming him or herself into an actualized balanced human being.

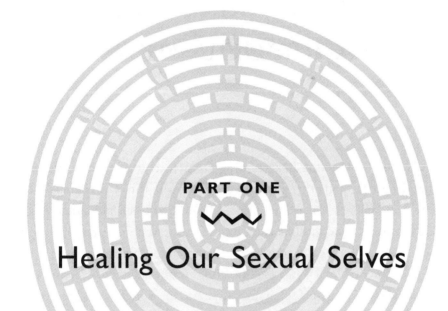

PART ONE

Healing Our Sexual Selves

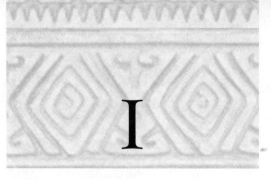

The Legacy of Quodoushka

I received the Quodoushka training from teachings given to me by Thunder Strikes and other guides in the Sweet Medicine Path in much the same way apprentices may have learned from their teachers centuries ago. The lineage of Quodoushka can be traced to traditions established over three thousand years ago from early Mayan and Olmec societies. While much of the rich legacy and the exact origins of the Sweet Medicine and Quodoushka lineage may remain a mystery, the wheels, keys, practices, and wisdom are still shared from teacher to student to this day.

It should be remembered that the sexuality teachings form only a small fraction of a greater body of knowledge called the Sweet Medicine Sundance Path of Turtle Island. These include healing techniques, philosophy, weaponry, law, martial arts, ceremonies, and rites of passage that honor our life transitions from birth to death. The task of accurately preserving the integrity of ancient teachings is formidable, and their survival frequently teeters on the brink of extinction. They must survive the ravages of vast cultural change and transcend the perceptions of countless individual teachers and students. While ancient knowledge naturally evolves through time, great care must be taken to keep its original intention intact. Quodoushka has survived and maintained its integrity due to the remarkable courage of the men and women throughout history who dedicated their lives to ensure this knowledge would be carried into the future.

Today, as in ancient times, students who wish to become Quodoushka teachers undertake many years of rigorous training through what are called Ceremonial Gateways. The process includes hundreds of self-reflection ceremonies that are designed to foster a deeper connection with nature and teach the skills needed for healing themselves and others.

THE EARLY SOURCES OF CHULUAQUI QUODOUSHKA

Hyemeyohsts Storm, in his book *Lightning Bolt,* writes one of the few accounts honoring the Zero Chiefs whose Medicine Wheel teachings inspired and guided the creation of many great cities of Mesoamerica, where these practices are said to have originated. While it is not within the scope of this work to detail the full spectrum of the Zero Chiefs' knowledge, it is helpful to understand the heart of their history as it relates to Quodoushka.

Zero Chiefs were highly cultivated warriors, healers, and teachers who established the legendary cities of the ancient Yucatan region that flourished with more than two hundred thousand people over many generations. Their profound discoveries in mathematics, agriculture, astronomy, and architecture, along with the Flower Soldiers they trained, led to the creation of vast and beautiful cities, whose governments were based upon equal representation of men and women. Their entire philosophy was dedicated to building communities that taught individuals how to live in balance, harmony, and self-freedom. One of their greatest achievements was the discovery of zero, which helped people relate and connect to what they could not see—the invisible world of Spirit.

Not all Mayan cities were utopias, however. Their history is stained with constant invasions and civil wars that decimated these early societies. Massive earthquakes, volcanoes, and droughts, along with generations of murder, pillage, disease, and greed, drove the Zero Chiefs underground. The history we read and the cities we know of are the stories of the victors. These societies, which were run by feudal warlords, kings, and queens, were ruled through governments and priests who propagated human slavery. Some cities practiced human sacrifice as a means to appease their gods and maintain the systems of the slave lords. None of these ancient cities survived. The teachings of male-female balance, freedom, and self-discovery were wiped out and outlawed. The Zero Chiefs, Flower Soldiers, and anyone who opposed slavery were hunted and slain. Some of the few who survived eventually migrated to North America.[1]

THE TEACHINGS OF TURTLE ISLAND

The fragmented ruins and artifacts of Chaco Canyon and Canyon de Chelly suggest survivors from these civilizations managed to preserve some ancient knowledge of astronomy and architecture. In 1250 CE in Oaxaca, scattered leaders and teachers gathered in council to assemble knowledge from those who had escaped the invaders. It is here that the Twisted Hairs Elders were named from what was called the Rattlesnake School of Turtle Island. During this time, a branch of teachings known as the Sweet Medicine Sundance Path of Turtle Island* was established. Members of their councils were named Twisted Hairs because their teachings of self-responsibility through the gateway ceremonies for personal evolution represented the braiding together of knowledge and wisdom from many traditions.

After the Spanish exploitation of Mexico, a relatively small number of women and men who knew these teachings escaped. They preserved and secretly taught the Wheels and Keys of Freedom. Knowledge that was once a full head of hair was reduced to a few strands. From the 1500s on, more catastrophic events, including epidemic disease, earthquakes, and wars with European conquerors forced further migration as the Zero Chiefs and Flower Soldiers traveled to join different tribes across North America. The brutal Indian Wars, along with Christian missionaries who sought to convert Indians of all tribes to conform to their beliefs, pressed

---

*Turtle Island is the name for North, South, and Central America, and includes the land masses of Australia and New Zealand.

what knowledge was not forgotten into absolute secrecy. Today more than 90 percent of Native Americans are various types of Christians, and most have never heard the teachings of the Zero Chiefs. Furthermore, descendants of many tribes deny that there are any sexuality teachings whatsoever within their great lineages.[2]

MODERN LEGACY

In 1992 Thunder Strikes became a Twisted Hairs Nagual Elder dedicated to recording and preserving the Sweet Medicine Sundance and Quodoushka teachings. Before this, in 1978, while Thunder Strikes was studying to become a therapist in California, one of his professors realized that Thunder Strikes had a significantly different understanding about sex. During the professor's class on male orgasms, Thunder Strikes demonstrated how to have a full-body orgasm using only his breath, without any genital stimulation at all. He was asked to give a presentation of the sexual teachings he learned from his grandmother and other teachers while he was growing up in Texas. His request to share the Quodoushka teachings with others studying to become doctors and counselors was granted by the Twisted Hairs Council of Elders. This began the modern workshop format of Quodoushka.

The Twisted Hairs Elders continue to see how urgently people need the teachings of freedom and self-responsibility to evolve and care for Mother Life. While Quodoushka and the Sweet Medicine Sundance Teachings are not a religion, they do present a way of living in balance and harmony with ourselves, life, and others. Understanding everything as an embodiment of both feminine and masculine energies joining in the sacred union called Quodoushka is a living tradition that continues to change and grow as people embrace it today. Whereas the cost of sharing this knowledge may once have led to banishment or death, the greatest risk today is silence. Whereas once these teachings may have belonged to one tribe or another, what matters now is that as many people as possible learn and use them to become better human beings.

Using the Wheels of Life

The task of preserving complex systems of knowledge was achieved by recording information using what are called Medicine Wheels, or Wheels of Life. The term *medicine* is used to convey the wheels' healing purpose, wherein each word and each position on the wheel is a code or a key that can open a door to new perceptions. They are considered sacred wheels because the words are not randomly selected; rather, they appear as Medicine Wheels because they have survived the tests of time and because they work. Looking at concepts on a wheel allows us to take in information as a whole; it causes us to consider the relationships between things and thus takes us beyond the limitations of linear thinking. As we use wheels to learn about our sexuality, they guide us to think in terms

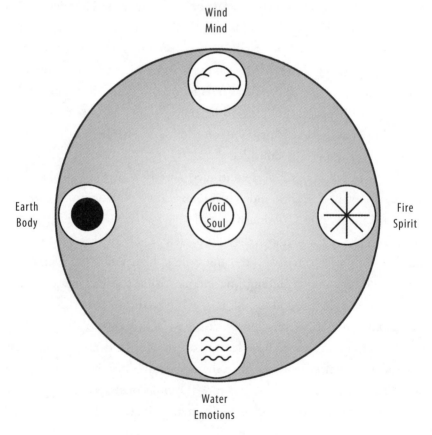

Wind
Mind

Earth
Body

Void
Soul

Fire
Spirit

Water
Emotions

Fig. 1.1. The Elements of Creation

of growth and evolution as we mature through the cycles of our lives. Do not let the simplicity of these ancient wheels keep you from experiencing their ability to activate powerful realizations inside you.

The Wheel of Elements lies underneath every wheel presented in this book. It describes the meaning of the cardinal directions South, North, West, and East. Other wheels include teachings on the noncardinal Southwest, Northwest, Northeast, and Southeast directions. South is the element of water and emotions, North the element of wind and the mind. West is the element of Earth and the body, East the element of fire and spirit. The Center is the element of the void and the soul. You may wonder why getting to know the function of the elements is so important to understanding sexuality. Consider that when we come together as lovers, the Wind of our breath quickens the Fire of our passion. The Water of our bodies' heat causes the Earth, our muscles, bones, and flesh, to come alive with pleasure. Any time we experience orgasm, we experience the element of the void, the source of creation through which everything is born. Remembering the elements of nature lays the foundation for feeling more connected to each other in our sexual experiences.

2

An Initiation into the World of Sexuality

*No matter how we are introduced to sex in our early years,
our first sexual experiences leave an indelible mark on our
character for years to come.*

PHOENIX FIRE WOMAN

It is said that within many native cultures, certain women and men specialized in the use of sexual energy for healing. Phoenix Fire Woman is a title given to a woman who is not only trained in the skills of lovemaking, she is acknowledged, by the community, as a medicine woman who is a wise teacher and a consummate healer. The same is true for a Phoenix Fire Man. One of the roles of these teachers was to ensure that young people were taught about the sacredness of their sexuality. They were first taught about how to carefully observe the forces of nature. When they were considered mature enough, they were shown how to approach sexuality with great care and were guided to treat the opposite sex with reverence and respect. For the most part, because initiating young men and women into the world of sexuality lies outside our culture's beliefs and is considered a taboo subject by many, the actual methods and accomplishments of

14

Phoenix Fire Women and Fire Men have remained secret. Throughout the following interview, I ask questions of a man as if a Phoenix Fire Woman had trained him.

Although this interview is hypothetical, comprising details from personal sources, it serves as a model for what an initiation with a Phoenix Fire Woman could be like. It speaks of the essential things a young man needs to learn and how he should be taught in order to become a mature, loving husband.

An Imaginary Interview

Amara: *Can you tell us how your training began?*

Adam: *When I was eighteen my grandmother, whom I will call Morning Star, brought me to Mary Fire Eagle's living room. I was introduced to six women and was asked to choose one as a teacher. Actually, however, my training began much earlier. Although I didn't know it at the time, my education started when I was seven years old learning about nature from my Clan Uncles, Neal Two Arrows and Edward Walking Bear.*

Amara: *What kinds of things did you learn from your Clan Uncles when you began?*

Adam: *They taught me that there was nothing I could perceive that was outside of me, but that it was a part of me only if I stayed connected to it. And of course the most important thing was to stay connected to Spirit, because this is the energy that created all the mineral, plant, animal, human, and spirit worlds. We never had any formal lessons on any of this. We went for walks, we hunted and fished together, or we hung out and talked.*

Everything that happened became part of the lesson. They tested my sense of seeing, touch, hearing, taste, and smell. They taught me hundreds of things about the land, flowers, trees, and birds, as well as fascinating things about the way human beings act. My real education wasn't about theory; it was about noticing, learning from everything. They taught me how to ask questions, how to observe, and how to listen. They encouraged me to be curious about life and to explore on my own. Once you learn to be more observant, you can take that into being with a woman. You perceive differently, because a woman has minerals, water, warmth, and breath, she has the emotional, mental, physical, sexual, and spiritual worlds inside her, and it was all created through the natural energy of spiritual sexuality. Looking back, I see now they were teaching me to refine my senses and hone my awareness. They were training me to be sensitive to reality long before I met Mary Fire Eagle.

Amara: *What were the most important things you learned from your Clan Uncles?*

Adam: *To feel the cycles of things. Years later I could take what I learned from nature and notice the changes in the smell, for example when a woman cycles through her moon (menstruation). All the changes a woman goes through, I could recognize, and I was able to communicate about them in much more responsive ways. As men, we have to be able to learn about these things, because "y'all are from Venus, and we're from Mars." We have to learn how to be able to get along and live together. Understanding things such as what a woman goes through with her cycles gave me a tremendous advantage when I became a man, because I understood better what to do about her changes. The most important thing I learned from my Clan Uncles is that a woman is closest to nature; she is nature, and she is natural. If you cannot align with nature, you cannot align with the feminine. Nature and the feminine are inseparable. This changes your whole perception of a woman.*

Amara: *Lets go back to your training with the Phoenix Fire Woman Mary Fire Eagle. Did your parents know about this?*

Adam: *Oh, yes, they asked my grandmother to arrange for my lessons. My parents trusted my grandmother and Mary completely and to this day have never asked me questions about it.*

Amara: *Did other people in the community know about your training?*

Adam: *Yes, there were certain people who knew, and there were other young men learning too, but mostly it was all private. There were young women too. They met with their Clan Aunts for many years, but I don't know exactly what they learned. There were no set times for these lessons, because we all had different levels of maturity and different temperaments. Everything depended on our talents and interests, and none of us had exactly the same training. My grandmother Morning Star oversaw our education. It was private because even learning about sex at eighteen is still considered forbidden by a lot of people. For the life of me, I don't know why, though, because this is probably the sanest thing I have ever done.*

Amara: *Tell us how you were introduced to the Fire Woman, Mary Fire Eagle.*

Adam: *As I mentioned, I was taken to meet Mary in her living room. I was asked to choose between six very beautiful women my grandmother selected for me to meet. Actually, my first choice was a gorgeous young red-haired woman who caught my eye immediately. I was totally smitten by her, and I fully intended to walk over to her, but for some reason I went to Mary instead. She was beautiful too, but she was thirty-nine, which seemed much, much older to me at the time. I am very glad I made this decision, because I know now it was a test that changed the direction of my life. All those women could have taught an eager young man plenty about sex, but it was Mary who became one of my greatest teachers. It was really Spirit that guided me to choose her that day. She taught me most of what I know.*

Amara: *How did you feel when you met her?*

Adam: *Awed. (Smiling and laughing) Loved. Accepted. Recognized. I never once felt uncomfortable with her at any time, no matter what the situation.*

Amara: *How did you begin? What kinds of things did you do together?*

Adam: *My first lessons were to see how what I had learned from nature could be applied to her and her body. For example, sensitivity of touch. She asked, "What part of my body feels like a rose? What part feels like a tulip? What part feels like a sunflower?" She had really rough feet, so her feet felt like parts of sunflower leaves. It sounds funny, but it was really quite innocent in many ways. We didn't just start having intercourse; that's really a misconception.*

Amara: *So here you are with a much older woman. What was it like for you?*

Adam: *Having a constant erection. It was endless! When you're young, sex is all you can think about, or at least that's what I thought about. The most important thing was the precautionary—no, a better word would be the sensitiveness of how you approach that kind of beauty, and of what it takes to partake of that kind of beauty correctly.*

Amara: *What kind of things would you do together?*

Adam: *I came over to her house many times. Sometimes her family was there too. We took walks in the woods; I worked in her garden and did things for her around the house. It was a better part of a year before we ever did anything remotely sexual together. The first part of it was my learning how to stay receptive while giving. I had to get over thinking about what I could "get" to satisfy myself. One day when we were in the garden, she said, "Touch my nipple. What do you feel, other than your erection?" So I learned to bypass the erectile function in my cock, and I thought,* Whoa, something else is producing the erection, not just her. It's her naturalness that's producing this, not just her. Now, how do you deal with this?

It was how she did things that was so amazing. She was very spontaneous, and she did all kinds of things to get my emotions going. At one point, I was feeling sorry for myself because I had to wait. I did everything I could to hide my impatience, but she didn't miss a thing. She would show me what was really going on in my mind, not what I wanted to make happen. What was happening was one thing; it was how I dealt with it that mattered.

The first sexual act was me performing oral sex with her. It was much later that we had any sexual intercourse.

Amara: *How did her husband feel about her lessons with you?*

Adam: *One of the most telling moments was something he shared at Mary's funeral. He said she had trained over a hundred young men to be real men. He was extremely proud of what she had accomplished. It's one of the reasons why I have never really understood jealousy. How can you be jealous when someone you love is learning and doing something that will give them more maturity, more sensitivity, and much more care about the world? How can you be jealous of someone you love who is getting that knowledge or that experience for themselves?*

Amara: *What were the things she taught you that affected you most?*

Adam: *It was learning through experience about what is natural, if you don't have all these taboos dumped on top of you on what sex is about. The most important thing was to be spontaneous. Spontaneity is the major approach of all sexual learning. Look at how often you plan something you think you should do sexually. What does that do? It automatically stops the flow of what's naturally happening. I also had to learn about the different anatomy types, which is one of the things you focus on in the first level of Quodoushka training. By being with different women and learning their sexual anatomy types, I came to understand a great deal about the natural differences between* *women—the sexual differences. Women are not all the same, and by coming to know their anatomy, you can be a much more caring partner, and you can satisfy a woman's needs and desires in a far more sophisticated way.*

Amara: *How did your sexuality training affect you as a husband later on?*

Adam: *My grandmother had a conversation with me before I got married. She laid down the law and said, "You better stay inside this." One thing was to never go to sleep on an argument without making love. Sure, Mary and her husband had arguments, and my grandparents did too, but it amazed me how quickly they came back together. They never went to sleep on an argument and always found a way to make love. My grandmother's advice has inspired me for over forty years, and it works. I haven't been perfect in my marriage, but it's not about being perfect; it's about finding the way to come back together.*

Amara: *After you married, you went to Korea. Can you describe the impact your training had on this part of your life?*

Adam: *I'd have to say these teachings are what brought me back home. While I was in Korea I met a man who was a healer and a shaman. At first I wasn't sure exactly whether he was a soldier or a farmer, but we soon discovered we had an unusually powerful connection. We exchanged many stories about healing herbs and such things. I was amazed how similar our backgrounds were. The last thing the he said to me before I left was, "When you receive two packs of Pall Mall cigarettes one day, you will no longer be killing, you will be healing."*

Years later, after many things happened that I won't talk about here, many horrible things during the war—I met with a medicine woman in New Mexico. I was totally disillusioned and sick and had forgotten what my early teachers had taught me. She said one of her Wolf spirit guides told her to bring me two packs of

Pall Mall cigarettes, even though she knew I smoked clove ciga-
rettes. Her spirit guides told her, "He will know what it means."
It was at this moment I remembered the shaman's words. The
cigarettes were a signal to wake me out of my despair. I knew I
had to forgive myself for the killing I had done as a soldier, and I
had to find the courage to heal myself.

   What does this have to do with the sexuality teachings I
learned as a young man? Deep down, for me, the courage of a
warrior, a lover, and a healer are one and the same. In the end,
sex is about reaching out to one another. It takes the heart of a
warrior to forgive, to heal our wounds, and to become a mature
human being. I think this is what my teachers were trying to
instill in me.

THE KEYS TO AN EFFECTIVE
SEXUAL EDUCATION

While it may not be feasible to turn back the clock to romanticize about
how ancient civilizations may have taught young people about sex, and
we may not have a grandmother or uncles so wise, it is possible to put
into practice the essential ingredients of a wise introduction to sexuality.
An initiation should begin years before anything sexual ever occurs. It
does not mean having early sex. In fact, an effective education emphasizes
patience and proper discernment, and it should encourage us to explore
safely. Above all, it should instill a strong sense of self-worth, responsibility, and respect. This requires careful guidance from someone who knows
us well.

   Without a caring mentor and clear principles, confusing messages
can take us off-course for years. Unfortunately, most of us receive little
direction about what to do with the strong sexual energy that awakens
in us around the time of puberty. In my case, when I was about fourteen
years old, my cousin and I went on a mutual date with a couple of friends
with the intention of fooling around, which we did. It was very innocent, and looking back, maybe a little too unsupervised. Nonetheless, it

was incredibly exciting to talk with and kiss a young man I barely knew. Fortunately, it was a positive experience—that is, until I shared my adventure with my cousin the next day. I was so thrilled to tell her how he unzipped my pants in the car, but before I could even finish my sentence, she shot back, *"You did what?"* I got the resounding message: I had gone too far, and I was certainly sorry I mentioned it to my cousin. I chewed on that guilt for a long time.

Although this experience did not deal a crushing blow to my adult sex life, it brought up the kinds of dilemmas that marked my explorations into the world of sex. On one hand, I could hardly think of anything else. I didn't even know what a hormone was, but mine were surging anyway. Yet, as I continued to explore my sexuality in a tentative fashion, every new experience brought up more doubts. What were my boundaries? What was too far? How did I know I could be safe? Questions like these come up for all of us during our early sexual forays, and unfortunately, because we don't know where to turn for advice, our initiations are filled with confusion, insecurities, guilt, and fears that take years to unravel.

Recently, while giving a lecture at a university addressing the topic of sexual health with nineteen- and twenty-year-old students, I asked how they got their sexual education. Out of fifty students, only two said they had any classes on the subject of sex since graduating high school. Like most of us, their real education came from whatever they picked up from their peers. Amid smiles and embarrassed laughter, there was a collective squirm in the room when I asked, "How many of you were taught that sex is something natural and good?" Their answers told me not much had changed since I was their age. Their formal sex education still consisted of clinical-sounding terms buffered by a reluctance to talk about what was really going on. Mostly they listed the things they were told not to do. While learning about the dangers of unprotected sex is important, it does not begin to address what is actually happening in the minds and bodies of students between the ages of twelve and twenty.

Unfortunately, the question of how and when to educate children about sexuality remains chronically vague, and there are no agreed-upon methods to effectively guide our youth through the changes of puberty. Are parents supposed to teach young boys and girls about sex with sincere answers to their concerns? Can schools or religious institutions effectively address the realities of sexual maturation without offending people's beliefs? Too often, the uncertainty about whom to trust and how we should educate our children leaves this crucial aspect of our lives up to chance. Without relevant and responsible early sexual guidance, we perpetuate unnecessary sexual difficulties again and again. According to Quodoushka, it is not only the reason why so many marriages fail, the lack of meaningful sexual education is the primary cause of drug addiction and abuse.

How is it that we require more instruction on how to drive a car than we teach our youth about the complexities of sex? How can adults safely steer a new generation toward enjoying a balanced and healthy life when our own sexual insecurities stand in the way? Clearly, the key is for parents, grandparents, teachers, and partners to become comfortable about sex themselves first. Whether we have children or not, each of us must seek to heal our own imbalances in order to approach sexual intimacy with greater wisdom and care.

Even if we have managed to enjoy many positive experiences along the way, most of us have entered into our adult relationships armed with almost no idea how to deal with the sexual challenges that arise. It has been said that the teachings of Quodoushka contain the missing links of meaningful education that should have happened for us around the time of puberty.

THE GUIDING PRINCIPLES OF QUODOUSHKA

What is most needed to establish a comprehensive understanding of our sexuality are clear underlying principles of law to abide by. Historically, indigenous people had little need for voluminous law books to address the minutiae of human behaviors. Their laws, which reach to the depths of human nature, are simple yet profound. While civil and social laws must change with the tides of culture, some laws are universally true, and thus sacred. There are two Sacred Laws of the Sweet Medicine Sundance Path that are the governing principles of Quodoushka teachings. The first

Sacred Law states, *All things are born of feminine receptive energy and are seeded by masculine active energy.* The second law states, *Nothing shall be done to harm the children.*

While these might seem hefty topics to introduce to young people, the meanings behind them are easy to understand, and they are demonstrated everywhere in nature. For example, how can seeds (masculine active energy) be born without first being placed in the earth (feminine receptive energy)? This law also applies to human behavior. Whenever we are receiving and open to learning something, we are expressing feminine receptive energy. Whenever we are making or actualizing something, we are expressing masculine active energy.

Understanding this law provides a clear way of knowing whether something you are doing is in alignment with nature or not. For instance, if we interfere with feminine energy by repressing women, obliterating a species, or damaging anything that can give birth, it stops the flow of creation. Harming the feminine principle interferes with conception and thus prevents things from being born. Likewise, interfering with the "seeds" of masculine creativity prevents the evolution of life. The word *seed* is used because ideas are the seeds of actions. The act of murder and the idea of greed for profit with no care for the consequences are seed thoughts that are against Sacred Law. These masculine and feminine principles are not about gender, for women can be greedy or can commit murder, and men can be open and receptive. Ultimately, this law states that for life to evolve in harmony, both feminine and masculine principles of energy must be respected and protected.

The second Sacred Law, *Nothing shall be done to harm the children,* means honoring the worlds of Grandmother Earth, including minerals, plants, animals, and humans. It also means to honor and protect "the child within." Introducing sexual acts to children is illegal in every society because it severely disrupts the maturation of a child's soul. Sexual abuse does so much harm to a child's spirit, it can take a lifetime to heal from the wounds.

PUTTING SACRED LAW INTO ACTION

A good place to start understanding the law of feminine and masculine principles of energy is by watching the beauty of nature. Years ago, an eight-year-old boy pulled me aside to have a private chat at a summer camp I was teaching. The furrow in his eyebrows told me he was clearly confused about something. Finally it came out that his friends were discussing sex, and he had no idea what they were talking about. There was no way he was going to admit he didn't know what sex was, and he was acutely embarrassed that he didn't know.

I'll never forget the way he went about asking me. He looked at a tree above us, whose leaves were shaking in the wind, to get to his big question: "Is kissing sex?" "Yes," I told him. "Kissing is one of the most beautiful things about sex. You see the way the wind and the sun are touching those leaves? That's like kissing. When your mom kisses your dad, that's the way they feel, soft and warm and fluttering like those leaves. Kissing is not the only thing that happens in sex, but it's one of the best parts, and it's very nice." The boy jumped up. The conversation was over. He returned triumphantly to his friends knowing just what he needed to know. I probably didn't answer all his questions, and I'm sure he didn't share our conversation with the boys, but for the time being, it was enough. It is said that nature is the best and the truest teacher. When sharing about the Sacred Laws, there is no need to ever use the words "feminine or masculine principles." The best way is to start looking at how nature "makes love" all the time and talk about what you see.

When a trusted mentor shows us how to observe nature, it's to teach about the way everything intricately depends on everything else. It is also a fascinating experience for young people to watch animals mating or giving birth. If they are directed to see these powerful times with reverence for life, it not only produces a sense of awe, it instills the message that sex is natural. All that we see and hear about sex when we are young, and the way we are guided to deal with our feelings, creates the foundation for becoming a kind and loving human being.

THE WHEEL OF PROPER PARENTING

Our approach to sex and intimacy is also greatly influenced by the ways our parents inspire us to learn. When we support the attributes of this wheel and help them thrive in a child, the result will be a healthy, reliable person ready to have mature relationships. As adults, we can also use this wheel as a way of "parenting" ourselves to become more sensitive, creative, and natural lovers.

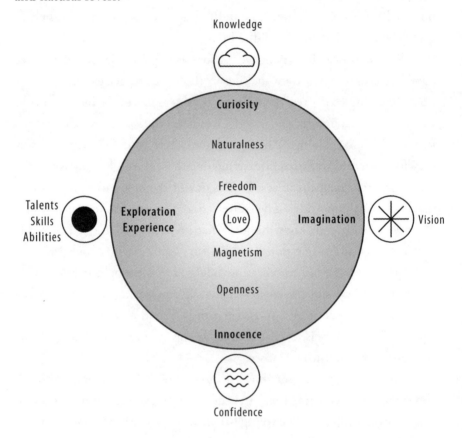

Fig. 2.1. The Wheel of Proper Parenting

The inner wheel describes the natural abilities we should foster in children from birth to puberty (about the age of twelve). The outer wheel describes the attributes that develop as a result, through the ages of twelve to eighteen.

South

Innocence Turns into Confidence

As children, before we are introduced to the idea that things are proper or improper, good or bad, wrong or right, we are free from guilt and the concept of sin. We are unacquainted with all the distinctions between things that we will later make; our perceptions are wide open, and we are full of wonder. Penises and vaginas are neither good or bad, they are simply rather interesting.

During these innocent, less complicated times, before we have any sexual experiences, we need to feel safe and protected. Yet when adults impose too many controls and adult perceptions about what is correct on us too soon, it represses our natural openness. When a child's innocence is properly protected and respected, the core of his or her intrinsic essence remains intact. When children touch their genitals, for example, they can be respected in a healthy way by allowing them to simply observe what they find interesting. Pretty soon their attention will move to something else. These initial moments of innocent wonder help us learn. When guidance is given in relaxed ways at the right times, it creates the ability to act with confidence. When our innocence is respected in our sexual lives, we can safely express spontaneous love and affection.

North

Curiosity Turns into Knowledge

Curiosity is the hunger to know. When moments of innocent wonder are encouraged, we have more and more questions. What kinds of things do we find fascinating? What escapes our grasp? The things that attract us tug at our minds and tempt us to find out more. Discouraging the desire to investigate leads to boredom, dullness, and rebellion later on.

I once read a story about a young man who did not want to do anything but fish. He happened to be in a school that allowed everyone to do only what they wanted to do, as long as no one was hurt. Students had to track down a teacher if they wished to learn mathematics, farming, or any subject. This particular young man took the idea to an extreme and spent over three years doing nothing but fish in a pond every day. The teachers and parents held fast to their idea that children learn best when they do only what truly interests them. When he graduated at the age of sixteen, he walked into a high-tech computer firm and landed a six-figure job without ever having used a computer. What happened? His mind was so fine-tuned to observing the way things function, he could apply its power to figure out anything. What looked like laziness on the outside was in fact years of the kind of study few of us achieve.

Of course, some of our curiosities lead to crashes and burns. We have all been hurt by our own and other people's blunders. Saying the wrong thing at the wrong time, transgressing boundaries, or having sex when we don't want to can make us wary of opening ourselves sexually later on. Yet we have to give each other and ourselves time to learn from our mistakes. The courage to stay curious is about remembering the power of how much we want to know. What was it like when we first touched a boy or a girl, or when we had our first kiss? What was it like when we heard our parents making love for the first time? Following the attraction of our curiosities is what gives us opportunities to gain the knowledge we need to become better lovers.

West
Exploration and Experience Turn into Talents, Skills, and Abilities

When our innocence and curiosity are respected, we naturally want to experience whatever we possibly can. To find out what works, and to develop our talents, we need some challenging adventures. Obviously, exploring doesn't end with childhood, and, in fact, whenever we let ourselves get complacent about things, the universe usually arranges some sort of drastic change to shake things up.

But it's the insidious ways we are discouraged from exploring that hinder our sex lives the most. Once while I was standing at the edge of pool with a mother and her three-year-old daughter, the little girl started throwing stones from around the deck into the water. I immediately lurched to stop her, but the mother signaled to let her be. She knew there was no need to interfere. My concern for her safety overrode what was actually happening; she was in no danger whatsoever. How often do we interfere with something our partner is doing because we want to protect him or her from harm?

Projecting our fears to try to stop our lover from exploring is an insidious habit that ends up destroying the very spirit of adventure we were attracted to in the first place. When we are afraid our partner may find something or someone more interesting than us, and we try to limit his or her experiences, the truth is we are in need of some new adventures ourselves. While the hunger to explore deeper spaces of sex inevitably comes with risks, it's the challenges we confront that give us the talents, skills, and abilities we need to be more intimate lovers.

East

Imagination Turns into Vision

When our innocent curiosities lead us to become more resilient through experiences, we gain the ability to imagine with power. Imagining our way out of sexual difficulties sometimes requires having a sense of humor. If we are plowing through the depths of despair and it seems as if hope is lost, do we have enough imagination to pull us through? How many different possibilities can we create? Can we persevere with our will, even if it means possibly dying while trying? This is what vision is.

When Chief Joseph stood on a mountain watching his people being raped and slaughtered, how could he say, "I will fight no more forever"? Faced with total annihilation, he had a vision that his true enemies lived inside him. He realized that he had to battle the enemy of his inner anger and hatred. In order to survive the unjust treatment of his people, as a true chief, he used the power of his vision to access the fire of his rage so that he could heal himself and bring hope to his people. A nation is a circle of power. Creating our own circle of power does not mean building a fortress of external protection so that bad things can't get us.

This story speaks of the futility of trying to escape the challenges that life presents. There was once a king whose soothsayer told him he was marked for death by the grim reaper. So off he went riding his horse to the furthest reaches of his kingdom trying to avoid his fate. Traveling to dozens of towns, he hired serfs to cover his tracks so that no living soul knew where he was. But as he collapsed exhausted and alone on the bed of a strange inn, he heard a knock at the door and was greeted by a cloaked man who smiled and said, "You're late! I've been waiting for you, and I almost missed you. What took you so long?"

Being overly serious is a curse to a good sex life because at some point, only our ability to lighten up and imagine something better will help us through. Lovers will leave us, perhaps even betray us, and our bodies will change. We will have to make our way through sexual droughts, and, if we are lucky, we will also enjoy many wild flurries of passion. Ultimately, it's the will to explore within our creative vision that can pull us through anything.

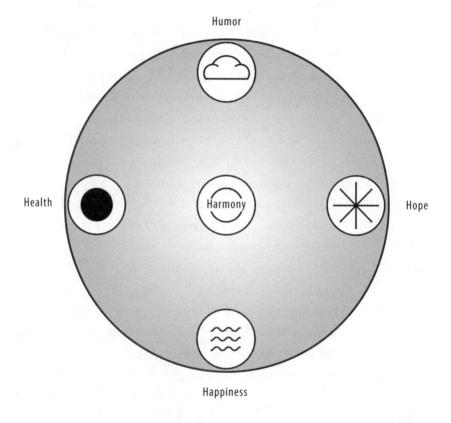

Fig. 2.2. The Five Huaquas

The Center

Naturalness and Openness Turn into Freedom and Magnetism

The center of a wheel is the catalyst, the driving force behind every direction around the circle. Love is the hub of the Wheel of Proper Parenting, because instilling love should be the underlying motivation behind all sexual education. Fostering a child's naturalness and openness allows a sense of magnetism and freedom to flourish. Inspiring, protecting, and encouraging our innocence, curiosity, exploration, and imagination in our early years gives us more confidence, knowledge, ability, and vision as adults. Keeping these qualities alive produces families and communities blessed by the Five Huaquas* of Health, Hope, Happiness, Harmony, and Humor. Ultimately, the foundation of a vibrantly healthy sexual life begins with how we care for our childlike natures.

*(pronounced Hoo-Kwah), the word *Huaqua* means "a gift of human experience."

3

Unlocking Sexual Conditioning

The point of the Quodoushka teachings is to experience sex as a natural expression, rather than as contrived and conditioned reactions to what others have molded and sculpted into our awareness.

Beyond lack of education, what keeps us from enjoying a rich and enduring sexual life? Where do the unconscious rules and conditions that cause us to hold back from sexual pleasure come from? Curiously, in this respect human beings are a lot like weeds. Even if we have been cut down to the root, the power of sexual energy is so strong we somehow manage to grow back through the cracks in the sidewalk. What if we could break free from the limiting conditions that no longer serve us?

As much as we might like to shrug off whatever holds us back from feeling the fullness of our passion, it is not an easy thing to do. Too often, negative messages become so internalized they limit us from feeling intense pleasure. Finding ways to enjoy a more richly satisfying sexual life requires looking more closely into the kinds of conditioning we have inherited. Once we see the ties for what they are, we can decide which conditions are useful, and which ones keep us from experiencing more than a small part of our full sexual potential.

There's nothing wrong with being molded into a turkey, unless of course you are an eagle in disguise. Although we may enter the world with an original essence like the high-flying spirit of an eagle, we soon forget where we came from. You can see the pure essence of what is called the Natural Self shimmering in the eyes of any infant. Having freshly arrived from the realm of formless Spirit, unencumbered by what it will soon need to learn, a newborn child has eyes with a glow so captivating we can't help feeling delight in its brilliance. In the shamanic view, being born into a physical form from the Great Round of formless Spirit is a remarkably rare opportunity to experience life in a human body. Soon, however, as this pure Spirit is trained to survive, the original essence of the Natural Self begins to fade. We inevitably forget we started life as bright and courageous spirits.

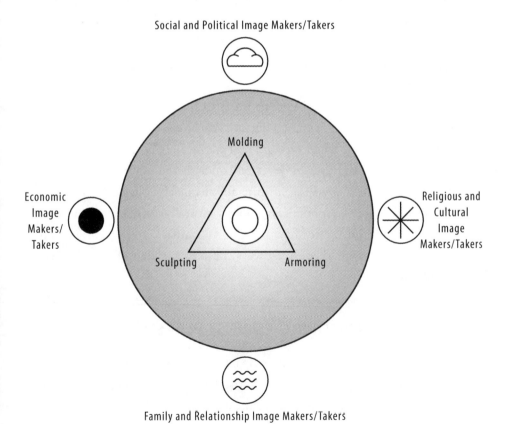

Fig. 3.1. External Image Makers/Takers

MOLDING AND SCULPTING THE NATURAL SELF

The instant we emerge from our mother's womb, the process of chipping away the Natural Self begins. As we land in the particular body, gender, and race generated from our parents' sexual energy and genes, the sculpting of the mold we were born into begins. Our first Image Makers are the people who train us to eat, move, react, and communicate. They begin the process of training us to become who we are supposed to be. The first years of our lives are completely focused on miming and mimicking millions of spoken and unspoken, conscious and unconscious messages from our Image Makers. Those who provide empowering models are Image Makers, whereas those who chip away our Natural Self with negative messages are called Image Takers. Our pure eagle-like spirit gets turned into a turkey, and whether we are aware of it or not, our lives are spent seeking experiences that remind us where we came from. Who were we before we were cast into a turkey?

Every time we make love, we have an opportunity to bypass all this conditioning. Moments of extreme sexual pleasure take us into "the time before," when our natural essence was still intact. Orgasms allow us to experience the source of the Chuluaqui sexual energy through which we were created. Even when our original nature has been shaped beyond recognition, crusted over by years of armor to the point where we may only vaguely sense anything infinite about ourselves, it's still there. No matter which racial, economic, religious, cultural, or physical mold we are shaped by, and no matter how parents, education, or events sculpt our awareness, our original essence always contains the seed of our immortal formlessness.

ARMORING AGAINST PLEASURE

Clearly, though molding and sculpting is necessary, it's also painful, because down deep we know our Natural Self is being sculpted away. To protect ourselves from this gradual, nearly imperceptible loss, we begin to armor ourselves against further pain. For example, when we first indiscriminately suck at food we want, we drool, smack our lips, smear food all over, and slobber. Pretty soon, however, we get the message that this is not okay. We get reprimanded, cajoled, and corrected until we eat properly. We don't like being scolded, so we start watching what others are doing, and we learn to eat like everybody else.

Along the way, we are trained to pay more attention to doing things correctly than to enjoying what we are doing. This is how we start to armor ourselves against pleasure. We block, become numb, and close down to pleasurable sensations in order to fit in, belong, and conform. The problem is, the armor we take on to avoid being an outcast also blocks us from feeling pleasure later on. Nevertheless, it's the turkey's job to stumble through, navigate, and decipher all these messages and to make sense of all this training. It's impossible to escape the molding, sculpting, and armoring that takes place, and perhaps forgetting our original essence makes it that much sweeter when we break through the mold, lay down the armor, and start feeling the natural pleasures of sex and intimacy.

Until then, usually we are so unconscious of all the conditioning we have acquired, we barely notice how we have picked up the habit of turning away from pleasure. Yet our resistance to pleasure shows in our stress and how seldom we choose sex as a way to replenish ourselves. Whether the conditions of our childhood were benevolent or violent, traumatic or mild, poor or rich, the challenge is the same. Will we remember our true nature and realize the preciousness of feeling alive, or will we squander the gift by staying a victim of our conditioning?

BREAKING THROUGH TO PLEASURE

Few would disagree that being held, making love, and being sexually passionate feel remarkably good. If sex is so marvelous, however, why do we so often let past conditioning rule what we say and do? Why do we frequently sabotage the very energy that could help us? And why, if we all have this pure essence residing inside, is it so hard to access and so difficult to feel?

To peer into the reasons why we let our past conditions limit our sexual expressions, Thunder Strikes has some wise advice. To begin with, asking why I did this or why this happened to me is not particularly effective. Asking *how* is far more useful. It's like asking why blueberries are blue or why is sex no longer exciting. *Why* questions are typically impossible to answer, and more often than not, the reasons take us in circles of fruitless explanations that only add to our difficulties. Asking *how* blueberries get their blueness or *how* our sex life loses its luster sets up a different, more neutral inquiry into the situation. Considering *how* things occur helps us gain the information we need to turn conditions around.

GETTING BACK THE ORGASMIC BODY

To explain how the original sexual forces that create us get trapped into a tight, restricted container instead of an open, relaxed, and naturally orgasmic body, it is helpful to think of life as a great movie. As we pick the locations, actors, dramas, and everything needed behind the scenes to create our personal history, do we see it as a movie? Are we the writer, director, and producer, attracting wise teachers, relationships, and lovers, or does everything that's happening make us feel like an extra? Are conditions turning us, or are we turning conditions into opportunities?

Turning Conditions Around:
The Unusual Sculpting and Armoring of Emily

A young girl in her early twenties came to a session of a Quodoushka workshop. She was quite attractive and seemed to have an unusually sex-positive background. She explained that her father was an erotic artist, and she grew up in a home where walking through the house naked was a regular way of life. For her, the conditions of her social upbringing taught her to feel completely comfortable seeing naked strangers. She said it was actually rather boring at times, and there were no instances of feeling threatened by abuse. She was the only person to raise her hand when we asked whether anyone had parents or someone in their childhood tell them sex was natural.

Nevertheless, the molding and sculpting of Emily's conditions created as thick a coat of armor as if she had come from a much more repressive situation. Despite her seemingly sexually free background, she was noticeably the most nervous, frightened woman in the room. Being naked was the most natural thing in the world; intimate conversation, on the other hand, was difficult for her. When participants were asked to share privately with a partner how they learned about sex, she broke down sobbing. What was a relaxing experience for everyone else, sharing intimate conversations with a person of the opposite sex was something she had managed to avoid her entire life. Although it was easy for her to be naked, and she had grown up in a mold of apparent sexual openness, she had armored herself against intimacy.

Gradually, throughout the Quodoushka workshop, Emily gently faced her fears and insecurities about talking to men. She turned her conditions around so that instead of being bound by what she grew up with, she found opportunities to change the story. She went home feeling safe to enjoy friendships with men without needing to be sexual at all.

Rex and Sonia:
Breaking the Mold and Resculpting for Pleasure

Rex and Sonia had an interesting upbringing. Both had parents who were important Malaysian diplomats. After receiving excellent educations at Ivy League schools, they later became surgeons. Rex grew up in a family that never showed public affection, and he had never seen his parents touching in any way while he was growing up. Rex and his three sisters were proof his parents had had sex at least four times, but, he added, "Any other evidence of intimacy was removed from sight." As a teenager, Rex attended a religious boys' school where his sex education consisted of secretly watching porn videos with his buddies in his dorm room. Bonding in these late-night meetings, he learned how men should behave with women—quickly pounding away to the finish.

Rex met his wife, Sonia, at the co-ed high school graduation prom and fell in love with her. Obeying the unspoken rule not to have sex before marriage, which had been instilled by family and peers, they soon married and had their first experience of intercourse. For the next ten years they created a lovely home together, started a family, and had highly successful careers. Unfortunately, as is all too common, although there was still a strong attraction between them and they clearly loved each other, their sex life petered out to nothing. They were friendly and busy but had no idea why the passion was gone.

Their story is an interesting movie with a common theme, the title of which could be "All Dressed Up with No Place to Go." Fortunately, this couple was determined to break through their molds, slice through the armoring, and reclaim their passion for each other. To add to the drama, however, a year before this scene, Rex had an affair. After going through the pain of betrayal, his lovely and rather wise wife forgave him. But she still could not bring herself to make love to him a year later.

To turn their sex life around, instead of harping on why this happened, they focused on sharing honest feelings and learning how to approach lovemaking differently. They realized that their sexual education hadn't progressed past high school and that they had never learned how to talk openly about their sexual feelings. Of course, sex became dull, and it wasn't anyone's fault.

While breaking through our molding, sculpting, and armoring is certainly difficult, it does not have to be a devastating, traumatic ordeal. For Rex and Sonia, learning how to communicate differently, as well as learning how to slow down and be more sensitive to each other's sexual desires, opened the door to forgiveness. He was touched by her willingness to forgive, and she was moved by his eagerness to find new ways to give her pleasure. Learning other ways to approach each other sexually created the possibility for renewed passion. Their story is still unfolding, and there are many more layers of conditioning for them to become aware of.

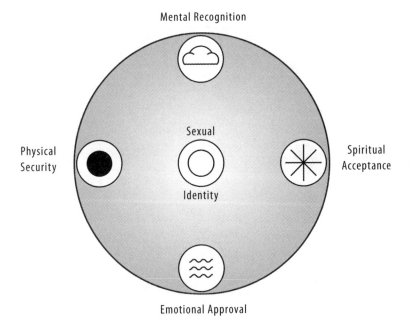

Fig. 3.2. Motivational Intent

THE DEEPER LAYERS OF CONDITIONING

How Emotional Approval Runs Our Sex Lives

According to the Twisted Hairs Elders, seeking emotional approval causes us to lose more energy than anything else we do. Seeking to be liked and loved is so ingrained into our behaviors we often fail to see how much needing approval from others runs our sex lives. Needing emotional approval is quite different from liking affection. For example, there is a huge difference between undressing in the dark because we're afraid our lover won't like our body, and disrobing seductively with the desire to arouse. In the first instance we're waiting for emotional approval, whereas in the second, we can enjoy being seen without worrying about what someone thinks.

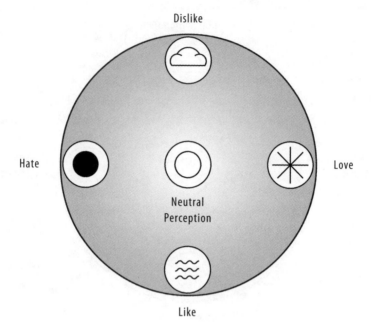

Fig. 3.3. The Five Human Perceptions

The Five Human Perceptions Wheel describes how we are motivated by other people's approval. Consider how much of what you say and do is actually an attempt to make sure someone likes or loves you. Sure, being complimented and getting affection is nice. It becomes a problem when the need for approval dictates your major decisions, and most of what you do is actually an attempt to be liked or loved. The teaching here is that we live in a wheel of five perceptions, where some people will naturally like and love us, while some will dislike or even hate us. Others may have a neutral perception, especially when they don't even know us. Accepting all five perceptions, and not taking them personally, is the key to reducing the vast amounts of energy we waste making sure we are liked or loved by everyone. This is especially useful in intimate relationships, when, for example, we want to make love and our partner responds with a neutral "Maybe later." The more we accept that at times we will have neutral responses, get rejected, or even be disliked, the less we will need to rely on approval from others.

FITTING IN, BELONGING, AND CONFORMING

Underneath everything, we bend and twist inside ourselves to satisfy our need for emotional approval, and what motivates us to keep the social conditioning of our Image Makers intact is the need to fit in, belong, and conform to what others want of us. Not fitting in, not belonging, and not conforming is so threatening, we will do things completely contrary to our natural inclinations. On a grand scale, it is easier to see the extents to which we will go to fit in with what others want us to do.

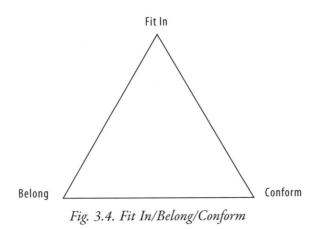

Fig. 3.4. Fit In/Belong/Conform

Conformity on a Grand Scale

A recent report of Catholic institutions in Ireland was made public after documenting over two thousand cases of severe physical, sexual, and emotional abuse of boys and girls. These were children placed into institutions from the 1930s to 1970s because they were accused of petty offenses such as truancy or begging, while others were abandoned orphans sometimes forcibly removed from single mothers. The study concluded that church officials encouraged ritual beating, failed to stop rapes and humiliation, and systematically shielded their orders' pedophiles from arrest amid a culture of self-serving secrecy. Victims were further burdened by an agreement between church and government officials to leave the offenders unnamed while offering partial financial compensation to the victims who came forward. The report states: "The harshness of the regime was inculcated into the culture of the schools by successive generations of brothers, priests and nuns."

In cases like these, where the government, institutions, congregations, students, teachers, and entire communities have a hand in perpetuating violent conditions for years, the need to fit in, belong, and conform has catastrophic consequences. In hindsight, it is easier to feel outrage and see the extent to which we will conform to prevailing conditions by turning a blind eye to endemic abuse. Yet the cost of fitting in, belonging, and conforming is enabled by how we, one by one, refuse to take responsibility in our daily lives for more personal transgressions. The next story is an example of how even well-meaning conditioning goes awry if it's too aggressively enforced.

Harsh Conformity

While visiting a Buddhist monastery, an ordained monk told the story of a mother who was banished from the community because she imposed basic Buddhist principles to an extreme. She raised her family forbidding her sons any contact with girls and made them adhere to obligatory practices of meditation, ceremony, and a strict vegetarian diet. Straying far from the Buddhist ideals of balance, peacefulness, and compassion, the boys became heavily addicted to drugs, quit their education, questioned their sexual orientation, and were unable to sustain healthy relationships. Years later, they were both welcomed as visitors, but the nuns and monks voted to ban the mother from the monastic community.

On a more personal level, the following story shows one of the ways we try to fit into relationships and compromise our autonomy.

Staying in Order to Belong

Jackie was a retired social worker. After working as a consultant, living on her own, and dating a boyfriend for several years, she met a man she really wanted to move in with. For about two years, their lovemaking took her into sexual places she had never known; she was mesmerized by his charm and infatuated by his potentials. Although he continued to court several women, as agreed in their open relationship, he assured her that she was the most important woman in his life. In time, as the other women fell away, she felt more and more wanted and desired by him. She felt secure and acknowledged for being a beautiful woman for the first time in her life. Plus, she had more sex during those two years than she had in all of her previous relationships.

Her need for emotional approval, in the form of being sexually desired, caused her to overlook the painfully obvious demise of their relationship. Friends started disappearing. Arguments and irritations that were once occasional became routine. What began as social fun escalated into heavy nightly drinking. For well over a year Jackie continued to downplay her boyfriend's increasingly strange behaviors with their friends and denied her own involvement with excessive alcohol. Sex was still good, and so she felt they would get through this phase.

Then he began to be physically abusive. But she reasoned she had quarreled too and convinced herself it was true, as he insisted, that she had provoked his anger. So she waited, overlooked the obvious, and hoped things would change.

Every relationship causes us to compromise some of our personal desires as we try to accommodate each other's needs. However, when the mainstay of a relationship deteriorates to the point where the security of belonging overrides everything else, things have to change. Fortunately, this couple got counseling and established new agreements to bring their relationship into a healthier place.

THE NEED FOR SECURITY, RECOGNITION, AND ACCEPTANCE

To add more intrigue to our movies, in the quest to fit in, belong, and conform, our sexual identity is formed by our deep cravings for security, recognition, and acceptance. First is the need to feel secure in our surroundings and physical bodies. Second, we crave attention from our friends, family, and lovers so that we can be recognized for our accomplishments. Third is the need to be accepted and believed in. The following story illustrates how one man turned around his need for security, recognition, and acceptance in order to have more authentic sexual choices in his life.

Gary's Hidden Identity

Gary worked for forty years on a family farm in Canada. Coming to a Quodoushka workshop for him was about as unlikely as becoming a prima ballerina: he had never been in a relationship in his entire life. Sex was something foreign, and although he seemed somewhat settled on his fate, after hearing a few of the teachings, he realized he did not want to remain celibate the rest of his life.

Gary's situation was unusual. Early in the workshop he shared for the first time that he believed he was gay. In his world this was completely unacceptable. No one in his community was openly gay, so he never acted on his feelings. Living by himself, his days consisted of working the machinery, managing the silos, and taking care of his elderly parents at night. Although he had considered moving to a city many years ago, his parents needed his help, so he stayed until they passed away. When a friend offered to pay for him to attend a Quodoushka workshop, he accepted without asking too many questions. He figured that since he knew very little about sex, it was something he should look into before he died.

We were charmed by his shy, friendly manner as he shared details of his life. It was the first time many of us had met someone his age who had never been in an intimate relationship. His situation put everyone else's difficulties in perspective, especially because he held no anger toward his parents, and he seemed relatively content. We welcomed him as a curious guest about to begin a new and wonderful journey.

Someone asked him what he missed most, and his answer was surprising: "It's not so much a relationship," he said, "or even the sex. What I really miss is being touched. Yes, I think that's what I miss the most, being held and touched by someone."

Who knows what messages this man received to live without intimate touch for so many years? In many ways, regardless of what we go through, it's how we play the cards we're dealt that matter. As this story shows, restrictive conditioning is not always filled with spectacular or dramatic ordeals; more often our social conditioning around sex is private and unassuming. The trouble is, we don't see that the ways we learn to protect ourselves from pain shut out pleasure too.

For Gary, expressing his need for intimate, loving touch was the beginning of an entirely new episode of his life, and thankfully, he decided it is never too late. Our need for physical touch is not an exaggeration. Without it we feel unbearably lonely, and we lose a sense of physical security in the core of our being. Gary was also recognized for being faithful to his parents, and while it was sad to see that he had waited so long, because he carried no bitterness or regret, he gained everyone's respect. In the end, though, it was his own self-acceptance that gave him the confidence to explore his sexual identity. It's a liberating experience to let go of all the extras that have no place in determining our sexual needs and desires. As Gary experienced, no one can see us for who we are until we start to accept ourselves.

A Ceremony of Self-Reflection
Nature Walk Talk

The Nature Walk Talk is a simple ceremony to help you reflect on your life. It is meant to heighten your awareness as you take a walk, ask a few questions, and listen to your answers. You may want to jot down the questions that follow and carry them in your pocket as a reminder.

During the Nature Walk Talk Ceremony, everything that surrounds you, including plants, the wind, or anything that catches your attention, may spark thoughts and memories. When you are alone in nature, your Natural Self has a better chance to peer through the veil to give you useful insights. All you need is to find a place where you can be by yourself. As you are walking, if a person comes by, notice how you automatically adjust what you are doing or thinking. When you are by yourself again, think about the people who made strong impressions on you while you were growing up.

> Who were your major sexual Image Makers and Image Takers?
>
> What were the negative messages you got from the people closest to you?
>
> What were the positive messages you got from them?
>
> How are these messages affecting your current relationships?

Simply let any insights you gain float in and out of your awareness. To complete the Nature Walk Talk Ceremony, thank yourself for taking the time to reflect in this way. Also thank your Image Makers for being a part of your life.

Sexual Choices, Sexual Preferences

Our sexual preferences and the types of relationships we form reflect the way our soul can best grow and learn. While our intimate partners are our best teachers, they are also our greatest tyrants, and the decisions we make about who to be sexual with are the most important decisions of our lives.

WHO TO BE SEXUAL WITH

Placing the various types of sexual preferences on a wheel sends a clear message: each one is a valid means to discover who we are. While the vast majority of people want to enjoy sexual experiences with the opposite sex, there are also those whose natural inclinations attract them to connect with same-sex partners.

West
Heterosexual

By far the most common preference is the desire to share sexual feelings with someone of the opposite gender. Like two poles of magnetic charge, attraction between two opposite forces compels us to come together. We gravitate toward heterosexual attractions not only because we can mate and raise children; we are also drawn to one another in order to know

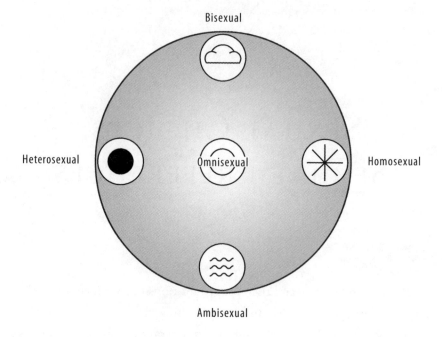

Fig. 4.1. Sexual Preferences

more about ourselves. This is because while we are born into one gender, we have both masculine and feminine qualities within our physical
and energetic bodies. Thus, when we have an attraction to someone of
the opposite gender, we want to know something about the less dominant aspect of our complete nature. As a woman, there is a part of us that
desires to connect sexually with men so that we can cultivate our creative,
masculine abilities. Likewise, men are attracted to women because it helps
them develop their feminine, receptive abilities. In this way, we grow by
looking into a mirror reflection.

East

Homosexual

This is the desire to know ourselves by exploring sexually with someone of the same gender. Most tend to agree that genetic, biological, and

environmental factors combine to create sexual preference. According to Quodoushka, an individual chooses to explore homosexual attractions as early as age three to nine years (or later). Quodoushka maintains that our sexual attractions are expressions of personal freedom. When we are attracted to someone of the same sex, we are seeking to learn through a like reflection.

In some indigenous cultures, homosexuality is considered a gift; and historically, many homosexuals held places of high honor. Homosexuals are referred to as "twin reflections" because they have the capacity to keenly understand the motivations and behaviors of both sexes. As a result, many are exceptionally sensitive individuals with refined sensibilities who frequently develop brilliant creative talents. Some people are born with strong homosexual preferences and prefer sharing sexual intimacy only with same-gender partners, while others may wish to explore same-sex attractions for brief periods.

North
Bisexual

A man or woman with a bisexual preference enjoys having sex with both men and women. At some point, nearly everyone has at least entertained the fantasy of having sex with someone of the same gender. Or they have felt a same-sex attraction and are thus what we call "bi-curious." Merely having these desires or curiosities does not make you gay. In fact, although most of us have a clear sexual preference for either men or women, this can change during the course of our lives. A young boy or girl, for example, who wishes first to explore sex with someone of the same gender may later discover he or she actually prefers the opposite sex. Likewise, a person married to someone of the opposite sex for many years may come to prefer being with someone of the same sex.

Those who gravitate to both sexes may go through periods of doubt while attempting to decipher their sexual attractions. It is not easy establishing relationships when there is a question of sexual orientation. Thus, bisexual people usually explore different types of relationships to determine what suits them best. When we allow ourselves and each other time to discover what we most desire, it is easier to find contentment and happiness with our true sexual preferences.

South
Ambisexual

A person who is ambisexual prefers having sex with someone of the opposite gender, but under the right circumstances, with the right woman or man, could enjoy a same-sex experience. Likewise, an ambisexual person may have a homosexual preference, but on the right occasion with the right person, he or she could enjoy an opposite-gender experience. Thus, being ambisexual means you *mainly* prefer having sex with one gender, but at times you could also enjoy the opposite. Being ambisexual is far more common than you may imagine.

Ambisexuality and bisexuality are probably the least understood of all the sexual preferences. This is likely due to the widely held belief that it is wrong to have more than one sexual partner at the same time. Yet how many marriages could benefit by seeking to understand and share feelings about sexual preferences? In many cases, when a woman or man experiences a same-sex attraction, it does not mean she or he would prefer a homosexual relationship. Repressing our sexual curiosity only compounds feelings of shame and guilt and ultimately makes it more difficult to know our true preferences. It is said that if we were allowed to explore in an environment without stigmas, being ambisexual would actually be a phase of natural maturation.

Center
Omnisexual

Being omnisexual means to feel a sexual connection to all the worlds of Grandmother Earth. It means we can have orgasmic experiences in nature, for instance, when we see a sunset or watch the stars shimmering in the sky. It means we literally have such a heightened state of pleasure while swimming, sitting on a warm boulder, or walking on a mountaintop that we experience a feeling of oneness with all creation.

While we can all have these omnisexual experiences—and ultimately, vibrating in unison with creation is our natural state—the reality is that we are seldom able to maintain this level of awareness. Furthermore, while some would like to claim they are omnisexual because they have exquisite moments in nature, it does not mean they can avoid human sexuality. Omnisexuality is also the realization of a sexual, orgasmic connection to all human beings.

TYPES OF RELATIONSHIPS

Along with the need to express our sexual preferences comes the desire to choose the type of relationship where we can best explore our attractions. Each of these relationship types has its challenges, and whether we are aware of it or not, we choose one form of relationship over another depending on how our spirit needs to evolve.

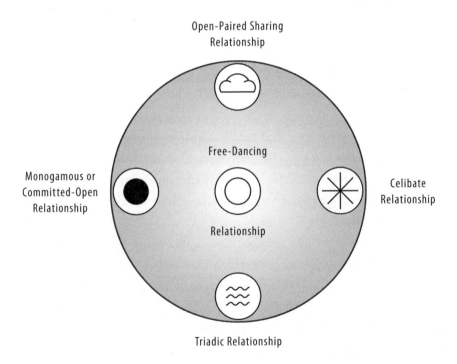

Fig. 4.2. Relationship Choices

West (option 1)
Monogamous Relationship

The Nagual Elders of the Sweet Medicine Path say that while a monogamous relationship can be the most fulfilling type of relationship, it is also the most difficult to sustain. Clearly, choosing to fulfill our needs and desires with a single individual requires a great level of commitment and maturity. Finding one person who will meet all our changing social, economic, intellectual, emotional, and sexual needs over the course of a lifetime is a monumental endeavor.

Monogamous relationships are considered by many to be the cornerstone of a stable society. Especially when it comes to raising children, the reliability and stability provided by having two loving and dedicated parents works best for most people. Monogamous relationships provide us with a place to open ourselves sexually and build our homes with the one person who loves, supports, and believes in us most. Furthermore, it's deeply fulfilling to share our dreams and defeats with someone we completely trust.

Promoting monogamy as the only acceptable choice, however, causes many people to feel inferior if they fail to find the correct partner to have a relationship with.

While remaining loyal and totally committed to one person can be extremely rewarding, it's not the only type of relationship possible. Those who choose this type of relationship must strive to ensure that emotional, mental, material, spiritual, and sexual necessities are satisfied for mutual benefit and welfare.

At various points in a monogamous relationship, it is common for partners to go through phases in which they feel as if they have stopped growing. One or both may question their feelings of attraction and wonder whether their compatibility will last. When partners choose to stay in a monogamous relationship, both must maintain the commitment to support and challenge each other to grow. While at times the sacrifice of personal freedoms may seem great, sharing enduring companionship with a beloved is profoundly fulfilling.

West (option 2)
Committed-Open Relationship

Although the benefits of monogamy are undeniably great, when individual growth is too limited, other types of relationships can be considered. One alternative to being completely monogamous is to establish a committed yet somewhat open relationship. In this type of arrangement, all the described benefits and challenges of monogamy are clearly defined between two people. To open the relationship in a limited way, at certain times, and with certain people, the partners agree that one or both may become intimate with someone else in clearly defined ways. For example, a married couple may decide to invite a man or a woman to join them for a sexual experience, or one partner may have sexual relationships in certain circumstances with other partners. The key to having a successful committed-open relationship is to ensure that the primary relationship is firmly established. There must be an abiding commitment to communicate honestly about all of your needs and desires in order to create agreements that work for both partners. (See my book *Sexual Agreements* for more guidelines on how to successfully create open relationships.)

South
Triadic Relationship

This type of relationship sits in the South of the wheel in the place of emotions, because the complexity of being sexually intimate with two other people often stirs up more energy than all the other types combined. The ongoing intensity of three people sharing sex and intimate feelings is exceptionally challenging. Triads require constant communication, and there is plenty of room for one person to feel left out.

Triadic relationships usually consist of two women and a man, or two men and a woman. Often, an established couple chooses to invite a man or a woman to join their relationship. In some cases, the woman wishes to have sex with two men, while the men may have no sexual desire for each other. In other instances, two men enjoy sex together, and the woman has sexual relations with both men. There are many combinations and variations depending on everyone's needs and desires. The triadic experience may be brief, or three people may choose to have a more lasting relationship. They may live together, or separately.

Though they are not common, I know of several successful triadic relationships in which children are being raised. This type of relationship can provide sexual variety, economic support, and sustained intimacy. If there is a stable and reliable environment, three people can combine their creative talents to create supportive families. Though they are often temporary, triads can provide expansive spaces for each person to grow and explore.

North
Open-Paired Sharing Relationship

In contrast to triadic relationships, which frequently form based on sexual attractions, open-paired sharing relationships are often created when two or more couples decide to share their resources. These relationships do not always start off solely because of emotional or sexual needs and desires. Frequently, economic considerations are the main reason to establish this type of relationship. Both couples see the advantage of sharing resources to raise children or to actualize careers and business.

As with triadic relationships, open-paired sharing relationships involve sexual complexities that create a dynamic that is not always easy to maintain successfully. However, I know of several open-paired-sharing, communal types of relationships where children are supported by the supervision of many caring adults. Although it can be confusing because their family is so different from that of their peers, the children I know who are raised in this manner often develop strong and resilient communication skills. While they sometimes miss the concentrated focus of two parents, they appreciate the mentorship that comes from having four responsible people committed to their upbringing.

Not all open-paired sharing relationships involve children. Some couples come together because they want to explore their sexual attractions. They may share intimacies for a brief or an extended period. In these cases, four people can enjoy the pleasures of sexual variety while creating lasting friendships and caring homes. When good agreements are established and maintained, this type of relationship can provide the space and support for visionary accomplishments.

East
Celibate Relationship

Sometimes the best choice is to be in a relationship with one's self. Quodoushka makes a distinction between celibacy and abstinence. Abstinence means to abstain from sex completely, whether by choice or default, whereas celibacy is a choice to "celebrate" our own sexuality. Celibacy is placed in the East of the Medicine Wheel because at times it can creatively expand our vision and passion for life. It is an opportunity to explore ourselves and this includes sexual self-pleasure.

Enjoying periods of celibacy, of refraining from sex with others for brief periods, can be rejuvenating and refreshing. Often, however, we are celibate because a relationship has ended, we don't want sex inside an existing one, or we can't find a partner. For these reasons, we are usually not happy about being celibate. We rarely choose celibacy consciously to restore our sexual energy or to reflect on our life's purpose.

When we are celibate for too long because we are disillusioned, afraid, or turned off from sex, it's not a healthy choice. On the other hand, choosing to be sexual by ourselves in order to reflect on our lives more deeply can be one of the best times of our lives, especially if we also cultivate the friendships and support we need. Then, when we are ready, and perhaps have acquired more wisdom, we can select the type of relationship where we can learn the most.

Center
Free-Dancing Relationship

On one level, free-dancing is what we commonly think of as dating. It means we are seeking a suitable person to spend time and possibly to have sex with. Sometimes we become a free-dancer after ending an intimate relationship; other times we choose to experience a variety of potential partners and are not ready to make a commitment to one of them.

Not all free-dancers are going through a temporary phase of seeking a life partner, however. Some may prefer having several long-lasting intimate sexual partners with whom they freely "dance" for their entire lives.

Today, with so many marriages dissolving, more men and women are becoming free-dancers later in life. It seems fewer people are willing to remain in unhappy relationships for years and years. Clearly, one of the main reasons why couples separate is to find greater sexual satisfaction. For many seeking companionship later in life, the dating rules have changed considerably. For one thing, sex outside of marriage is more acceptable than it was in previous generations and it is rarely an embarrassing stigma to have had several wives or husbands. Most significantly, the Internet has dramatically shifted the way free-dancers go about looking and connecting with potential mates.

It wasn't that long ago, for example, that a lot of couples would have been reluctant to admit they met through an online dating service. Over the last few decades, the Internet has outpaced all other methods people have used in the past to find partners. It used to be that the number-one way people in this country met were through church-related functions. Now, more people meet through the Internet than in bars, social groups, and all church functions combined.

While meeting someone online may not be the way you choose to find a mate, one thing seems constant: being single is certainly an adventure. Whether this period of exploration is brief or lasts for years, the desire to bond intimately is a powerful drive that carries us through the attempts, rejections, and also the beautiful experiences that happen while seeking an intimate partner. Above all, it is important for free-dancers to let go of agendas from the past and enter new relationships with clear intentions.

Free-dancing can either be a period of loneliness and longing, or a time of great personal growth. If we use it as a time to improve ourselves and to experience the kind of intimacy we would like to have, the care we take during our dating adventures can lead to far more satisfying and fulfilling relationships.

All of the exercises, ceremonies, and teachings of Quodoushka can be used to gain clarity about our sexual relationships. Whatever kind of preferences we have and whatever type of relationship works best for us, there is no question the sexual decisions we make are amongst the most important opportunities of our lives.

DESIGNING SEX INTO YOUR LIFE

When our relationship choices are clear, everything is working, and life seems like a series of green lights, finding opportunities for sex is not that difficult. The real reason we do not enjoy our full sexual potential has nothing to do with having enough time or meeting the right person—it's a matter of using our internal energies correctly, in harmony with nature. Going against the grain of how we are designed to function dissipates our essence and causes us to lose our health. Turbulent emotions and mental fogginess exhaust the physical body and drags the spirit down. Like

RECEIVE WITH CARE
by teaching one another with respect, honor,
and dignity that Everything Is Born of Woman
and Do Nothing to Harm the Children.

HOLD AND TRANSFORM WITH INTIMACY by caring for our physical and one another's physical spaces.	**CATALYZE WITH SEXUAL ENERGY** by being intimate with one another.	**DETERMINE WITH PASSION AND LUST** by sharing with one another our fire, our inspiration, our spiritual visions.

GIVE WITH TENDERNESS
our e-motion, energy-in-motion,
freely flowing, expressing from
our heart space.

Fig. 4.3. Balanced Choreography of Energy

billiard balls hitting each other, one trouble leads to another until our lives become scattered, listless, and ineffective. There is no way we are going to enjoy a satisfying sex life when we are out of alignment with the natural laws of energy movement.

The universe models balance and harmony everywhere, even in the midst of seeming chaos. A tsunami, for example, looks devastating from our perspective, yet strong storms, like strong emotions, are simply different expressions of energy. While we may not be able to completely define harmony, evidence of the invisible "As above" forces that generate order are mirrored in the "So below" visible realms of existence. Earth rotates regularly on its axis around the sun, creating light and darkness while the planets and their moons revolve around the sun, just as negatively charged electrons orbit the positive nuclei of atoms. Energies within our bodies, including hormones, blood circulation, and sexual secretions, collaborate in fantastically complex ways. Harmony is the interconnected choreography of all these systems. Though our eyes may not see the underlying forces that govern the movement of Earth or our bodies, we certainly know what it feels like to be out of balance.

Whenever chaos throws us off and we lose strength in our intimate relationships, it is always because we are misusing the five human aspects of our emotional, mental, physical, spiritual, and sexual energies. This wheel shows how we can regain our equilibrium in the middle of anything. It can be used to understand the dynamic interplay of all appearances in the universe, including the internal and external worlds of experience. Here is how it works.

THE INNER AND OUTER WHEELS

In their abstract meaning, the elements shown in the inner part of the wheel symbolize all substances or phenomena, and they contain qualities displayed by their inherent functions. In other words, water flows, earth nourishes life, wind changes direction, and fire expands. The central element, called the void, is the original source from which everything comes and goes. The corresponding human aspects along the outside of the wheel are the emotions, physical body, mind, spiritual and sexual energies.

These are the correct ways to use our internal energies: Like flowing water, we are designed to give with our emotions. Like the nourishing minerals of Earth, we hold and transform energy in our bodies. Like the changing wind, we are meant to receive with our minds. The fire of our spirit expands and determines. Our sexual energy catalyzes everything else in our lives. By understanding how these elements are designed to function within us, we can avoid unnecessary loss of vitality and correct imbalances.

Center: Void
Catalyze with Sexual Energy

Our sexual-soul-force energy relates to all forms of intimacy, including sensuous touch, conversation, and creative endeavors, as well as intercourse and direct sexual play. Whenever we are doing what we love and are being creative, we are expressing an aspect of our sexual-soul-force energy. Catalyzing with sexual energy means to bring our sensitivity, excitement, and orgasmic passion into whatever we do.

Quodoushka places sexual-soul-force energy in the center of the wheel because everything we do is affected by the way we approach sex. The way we dress, the jobs we choose, the friendships we form, the things we buy, the homes we create are all in one way or another reflections of the role sex plays in our lives. Yet most of us design our days as if sex is an extra bonus—something to fit in when we can find the time. Without outlets for creative sexual expression, it's as if we have a hole in our center that weakens the strength of the entire wheel. When we ignore it for too long, it's as if we have a flat tire. Emotions erupt, and the mind becomes agitated and indecisive. The body gets sluggish, and our spirits sink. The improper use of sexual energy not only diminishes life's joy; it leads to psychological and spiritual perversions.

We also disturb a balanced choreography of natural energy whenever we rely on sex too much. Being obsessive, including brooding about how we are not having sex, leads to as much dysfunction as relegating sex to the back burner. Finding the proper balance and correct use of our sexual energy is one of the primary teachings of Quodoushka, because when we are in harmony with nature, we are meant to embrace the complete wheel of human experience.

This means we must learn to honestly communicate our heartfelt sexual needs and desires. It does not mean we should demand sex whenever we want it or withhold sex whenever we don't. These are examples of how we are giving (demanding) or holding sexual energy rather than catalyzing our life force energy with honest heart-to-heart communication.

There are many ways we can invigorate our lives by expressing our sensuous, orgasmic passion. Creative outlets alone, however, do not fulfill the human need for sex. To harmonize with the Wheel of Creation, we need to share our creativity and have actual charges and releases of sexual energy.

South: Emotions
Give with Tenderness

When we are in balance and harmony, we naturally give with tenderness. Yet most of the time, we do everything but this. Instead, when we give, we want something in return. We give but then resent having given. We give thinking we don't want anything, but then if we don't like the way we are treated, we say, "I gave so much, but I am not respected."

It is said that giving ends with the act of giving. When a lemon tree gives us one of its fruits, it doesn't stand there asking for water. Giving with tenderness means to give without any expectations. But how do we do this?

Emotions sit in the South of the wheel with the element of water, because our emotions function like various kinds of rain, dew, ice, mist, oceans, thunderstorms, and waterfalls. The many forms water takes correspond to how we change from feeling happy, anxious, sad, thrilled, or angry in a matter of seconds. Like water, which takes the shape of its container, emotions constantly change according to our situation.

Our emotions are designed to be fluid like water, and throughout a single day, we will naturally shift from one emotion to the next. We cannot always be cheerful any more than we can stay stuck brooding with envy, hatred, or a desire for revenge. However, it's the excessive roller coaster of moodiness, fear, anger, sadness, and depression that causes us to lose tremendous amounts of energy throughout our lives. The question is, are we like a boat tossing and turning with each crest and fall of our moods, or can we tap into the deepest essence of water to regain our equilibrium? How can we allow the full range of our emotions to move without being overrun by them? The answer is to give with tenderness.

Even anger and irritations can be expressed with kind regard for what another person is feeling. Debilitating outbursts of anger and stockpiles of resentment can be avoided if we express emotions more often. Rather than holding them inside until they turn stagnant, or letting jealousy and grievances about things people have done keep us perpetually off kilter, the secret to a balanced life is to focus on having more outlets to give. This does not mean complaining to anyone who will listen; that would serve only to fester and boil our feelings into a bitter bowl of congested, stale emotions. When we do this, it means we are actually determining with emotions—that is, we stay fixed in our feelings that we are right and the other is wrong. We forget how to give tenderly, especially when it comes to sex.

Unbalanced Choreography:
Elizabeth and Matthew

One day while they were making love, Elizabeth's lover, Matthew, turned his head away in the middle of an embrace and said he did not like the way she kissed him. It hurt her feelings in the moment, but she couldn't say anything (holding with the mind). Instead of giving with tenderness, and honestly saying she felt hurt, she avoided kissing altogether (determining with the body). Her boyfriend forgot all about the comment, but he started to complain about her lack of interest (determining with the mind). What came out later was an intense outburst of unrelated criticisms, all stemming from Matthew's comment about the way she kissed.

Most of the time, the breakdown of a balanced choreography starts with holding small emotional resentments and, as this story illustrates, quickly spreads out to the rest of the wheel. Instead of receiving with the mind, we mentally hold onto negative comments. Rather than opening ourselves to sexual intimacy, we determine to physically shut down our bodies. If we close off sexual feelings, our spirit sinks further, and we cannot find a way to catalyze or change the situation with heart-to-heart communication.

Often, when imbalances compound and we cannot trace the source, the best place to start is by finding a way to give. The key to giving with tenderness is being honest first with ourselves and then with others. Honesty melts away emotional resentments and gives us the time to rebalance our minds, bodies, and spirits around the wheel. While ending all conflict between two people may be too lofty a goal, the practice of giving with our emotions is a remarkably effective way to restore harmony, especially when we take this idea to heart in our intimate sexual exchanges.

North: Mind
Receive with Care

Continuing the Story

Elizabeth couldn't let go of that one comment, and she was making Matthew pay for it by withholding sex. No matter how hard he tried to say nice things, the words were lodged in her brain.

This is an example of how we can't get back to harmony because we are holding and determining with the mind instead of receiving with care. In many ways, the mind is designed to function like a camera, taking snapshots of whatever surrounds us. When we are operating in harmony with nature, the brain is meant to receive all the images we encounter. The trouble is, we are constantly distracted, and we don't know what to do with the deluge of information. Mental stress comes from overdosing on stimulation and having to decipher and judge the incessant stream of incoming data. Instead of carefully receiving the messages we need to pay attention to, we take on much more than we actually need to think about.

But narrowing the intake of information is not always possible or correct. Sometimes we need to care about disasters across the ocean and feel concern beyond our own front door. As technologies make it easier to inundate our minds unnecessarily, they also help us realize that even our most personal choices affect people we will never see. The challenge is to receive with care. The real issue underlying mental stress is not the volume of information we absorb, it's the way we misuse our minds with false thinking. It takes a minimum effort to neutrally perceive a situation and allow it to float by like a moving cloud. What bogs us down is when we cling to ideas and filter what's happening with unrelated interpretations. Instead of letting thoughts come and go, we fixate our brains on what we are making up.

In fact, we seldom see people or situations clearly, and we consume our energy by projecting what we think is happening. Buddhists call this "placing a head on top of a head." The story of two celibate monks on a pilgrimage beautifully illustrates the tendency to clutter the mind with pretenses and projections. One day while crossing a stream, two monks met a beautiful woman in distress who could not get across the running water. One monk immediately picked her up, took her to the other side, and continued his hike. The other monk followed behind, put off by his internal tirade. Finally he said to the other monk, "Why did you pick that woman up? You know it is strictly forbidden to touch women." With a perfectly calm mind, the monk responded, "I put her down an hour ago. Why are you still carrying her?"

Nowhere is the tendency to predetermine outcomes and place projections on top of what is happening more treacherous than in our sexual lives. We cannot feel or listen to our partners because we have seen them a thousand times before. We react to our internal dialogue and already know what they will say or do. Until we drop the false projections and already-made assumptions of our minds, we will continue to see only what we want to see and hear only what we want to hear. The key to clearing the mind is to slow down and pay attention to what is actually happening. Especially as a lover, there is always the opportunity to pause, appreciate, and receive with a spontaneous, caring mind.

East: Spirit
Determine with Passion and Lust

Continuing the Story

After being honest with herself about how much that one thing her lover said long ago had hurt her, Elizabeth finally realized that until she forgave him for his careless criticism, there was no way she was ever going to be able to fully express her love. Matthew did not know she had been hiding these feelings and had no idea why she kept turning away from sex. He thought he wasn't attractive enough. In the end, they saw how they were both making things up that were not true. Their talking ended with tender affection and opened the way for many beautiful sexual times to come.

In this story, it isn't until Elizabeth and Matthew let go of their attachments to the past that they can go beyond the limits of their calculating minds. Getting to this place, however, isn't always easy. If we are not meant to use our minds to determine what we want and what we don't, then how do we decide what to do? The answer is to determine with our spirit.

What is spirit? It may manifest as an internal energy that urges us, sometimes against all reason, to keep going despite countless setbacks. Other times, our spirit senses danger, so we decide not to do something. In reality, though we may call it a gut feeling, instinct, or intuition, we are often using spirit to determine where to go, whom to get closer to, when to act, and what to avoid. Spirit is the energy that propels a man to pull a child from a car that is about to burst into flames. He doesn't think about his own safety; he does what needs to be done. This is the fire of our spirit determining with passion and lust for life.

The energy of spirit is what keeps us from stealing from others. It's the internal force that drives us to learn new things and explore unknown territory. It's what moves us to meet a new lover after a devastating breakup. It is also the part of us that knows we are completely responsible for our every word, thought, and action. Every time we say yes to sex, and we mean it fully, we are listening to the inner voice of spirit.

Yet we frequently disregard what our spirit seems to be telling us. Like fire, our spirit can leap, expand, and grow unpredictably. It can be felt as internal warmth, for when we know something will help us learn, it is our spirit that is attracted like a moth is to flame. Just as strong emotions or mental assumptions pull us off balance, our spiritual determinations are not always correct. Too much enthusiasm and over-reliance on signs that we interpret as being correct can create misfortune. We can misinterpret spirit by getting too fired up by a possibility and then fail to notice when circumstances change. Too much of a fiery spirit is as dangerous as a listless one. The most common way we misuse spirit is to doubt our intuitive knowing. A charismatic person might try to convince us he or she is a great healer, but when we overlook dishonest, selfish actions, thinking we are listening to spirit, in reality, we ignore all the signs of deceit. In cases like this, we are receiving instead of determining with our spirit. We have a distinct sense that something does not feel right, but we go along anyway.

When our spirit is weak, nothing seems to really interest us, and we get bored easily. Even sex seems like a hassle. Typically, the last thing we feel like doing is melting into someone's arms. The way to strengthen our spirit and rekindle the flames of our passion is to get busy, do something creative, and give something to others. Then our spirit can say yes to sexual opportunities more often.

West: Physical Body
Hold and Transform with Intimacy

Sooner or later, all the imbalances of our choreography show up in the physical body. The body, and thus our health, is the most accurate gauge of whether we are disrupting the natural course of energy movement. This is why the Grandmothers of the Sweet Medicine tradition say, "The physical is it." Much the way Earth gathers sunlight and then radiates heat, when we are functioning in harmony with nature, we hold, store, and then transform the nourishment we take in. The key is to hold and transform energy with intimacy. This means we must *listen* to what truly nourishes the physical body.

Most of us have some sense that good food, consistent exercise, and proper rest are the major ways we maintain and restore health, yet we frequently overlook our sexual needs. Rather than value sex as an essential physical requirement, we often treat sex like a bonus and place it on a shelf labeled "Later." Furthermore, instead of focusing on ways to satisfy our basic needs for sex and intimacy, we exhaust our bodies and try to compensate in other ways.

Our overall choreography is skewed to the point that we have lost touch with what we actually need to stay healthy. Typically, we want too much stimulation, and we store too little sustenance. Strong emotions and mental cravings block us from knowing when we are truly hungry or how much sex our body requires. We usually notice that we are way off balance when something goes wrong in a major way. Artificial time constraints, and our approach to the many obligations we take on, produce the constant stream of stress that underlies all physical disease.

For example, if a woman has a disorder in her emotional energy, say extreme anxiety, it may manifest as problems in her menstruation. She may have severe cramps, headaches, or irregular cycles. In extreme cases, people fail to notice huge tumors in their bodies. Instead of learning how to sense the body's subtle signals of imbalance, we depend on the advice of others more than our own awareness and thus perpetuate poor health without realizing we are perilously teetering on unsteady ground.

When our overall choreography is off, leading a stable, healthy life is considered less important than gaining fame, possessions, and accomplishments. But we can lose our way and suffer misfortunes even in the midst of great success. It is only because we violate the natural equilibrium of the body's energy network that we require ways to restore harmony with our original nature. Neglecting the proper use of our emotional, mental, physical, spiritual, and sexual energies leads to rapid aging and lack of contentment. The cure is to establish a proper choreography of energy by remembering to give with tenderness, hold and transform with intimacy, receive with care, determine with passion and lust, and catalyze our lives with sexual expression through open heart-to-heart communication.

BECOMING A BALANCED HUMAN BEING

Acquired, Potential, Evolutionary and Creational Principles of Awareness

Becoming a balanced human takes us through the stages of acquired, potential, and evolutionary awareness. Until we sift through what we have accumulated from others and express more of our naturalness as men and women; we will never discover the beauty of evolving into our full feminine and masculine potentials.

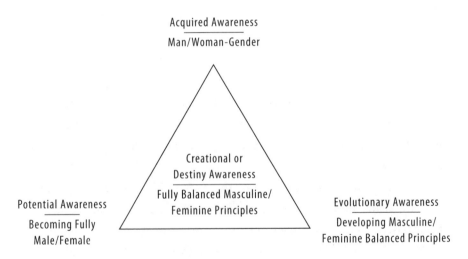

Fig. 4.4. The Evolution of Awareness

Acquired Awareness: Man and Woman

When we operate from our acquired awareness, our relationships are mostly about vying for positions of power in order to assert physical, economic, or psychological control. We spend much of our time struggling for our needs, wants, and desires to be met. Whether we take the dominant role, submit to constraints, or rebel against them, our lives are marked by an undertone of restlessness and lack of contentment. When we are operating from acquired awareness, we hold fast to the identities we have built up as men and women.

Within the confines of acquired awareness, which includes all the ways we learned to cope and survive in reaction to others, we play out endless battles over who is right. The macho man tries to dominate the subservient wife, or the female go-getter tries to assert her independence. It can also be turned around so that the man is subservient and the woman dominates. Regardless of who holds the position of power, even through we try to connect sexually, when we oppose each other with our acquired awareness as men and women, our separate agendas make it impossible to bond in mutually fulfilling ways. Orgasms are selfish to the point where each is more interested in what he or she can get rather than what can be given. In the struggle to evolve, grievances about trust come out as complaints and criticisms that preoccupy our thinking.

Men at this level of awareness are called "seed droppers" because they are busy carelessly spreading their "seeds" around. Seeds represent physical semen along with words and actions. Men at this stage do not want to take responsibility for the reckless, incomplete, or unconscious seeds they drop, and they resent feeling trapped. At this more selfish stage of awareness, men battle with their sexuality. They lack sensitivity and are either hungry for sexual experience or generally shut down. In their haste to get what they want, they cannot foresee the consequences of their actions. When a man is caught in acquired awareness, he is alternately driven by excessive desires and strong denial of his sexual feelings.

Women are called "egg carriers" at this level of awareness because they are overly compliant and do not properly care for what they conceive. As egg carriers, women conceive or carry things inside while they are taking shape. "Eggs" refers to the potentials of things, including children, homes, careers, and ideas. Operating within acquired social and commercial expectations, women end up resenting the burdens they have consented to take on. Sexually, women at this stage struggle to express their sexual passion. They may go through bursts of free expression, but then guilt creeps in and causes them to avoid sex. Women operating within the limited aspects of their acquired awareness are unclear, confused, and unsure about what they want.

At this level of awareness, women crave to bond in relationships. They want boyfriends, children, and homes as forms of security in order to validate themselves, but they do not properly care for what they bring forth. In other words, they get overly attached to relationships, things, or children but then feel burdened and thus blame external conditions for their predicaments. Any woman can be an "egg carrier" and any man can be a "seed dropper" whenever he or she acts without taking responsibility for his or her words or actions.

It should be kept in mind that these stages of awareness have little to do with a person's physical age, and they do not unfold in a straight, steady uphill climb. The truth is, we can have a wise, kind, or selfless moment of awareness in one breath, only to slide selfishly into the next.

Potential Awareness:
Fully Male and Fully Female

Moments of potential awareness happen when we get tired or bored with the status quo and something has to change. When passion, enthusiasm, or great sex starts to fade, the real work of awareness begins. During transitions from acquired to potential awareness, the motivations and desires that were holding careers, relationships, and families in place no longer work they way they used to. This is because when we are seeking our fully male and female potentials, we are no longer interested in the old molds and roles we created. In fact, the progression into potential awareness always includes the collapse of something; or, in some cases, it feels like the loss of everything. When we are moving between acquired and potential awareness, we often need dramatic upheavals to push us to grow. As we become more at home in our female and male potentials, we continue to make incremental, gradual shifts of awareness and we begin to learn through pleasure.

The early stages of potential awareness are marked by periods of sexual frustration and dissatisfaction. If we resist discovering our female and male potentials by holding onto old needs, wants, and attachments, we either shut down sexual feelings or we lash outward in bouts of anger. We know we want to be free from something old, but we don't yet know what we truly desire or need. What we used to want so much we no longer care for, but the new motivations are not at all clear. We still slip back into our acquired awareness where dishonesty, betrayals, lack of interest, and a kind of sexual distance that is difficult to communicate about sets in.

Entering the territory of potential awareness can be quite disorienting. Whether intimate feelings change gradually or suddenly, leaving behind the things we desired as partial men and women rarely happens peacefully. Nevertheless, in potential awareness, although we may try to sweep our new desires under the carpet to try and hold onto relationships or possessions, sooner or later the need to experience a different kind of awareness shows up.

Breaking through into male/female awareness can appear as depression, desperately trying to find a partner, divorce, or extended periods of listless boredom. Curiously, it can also happen at the peak of great achievements. At some point, when we are entirely fed up inside the limitations of our acquired awareness, things finally come to a head. Though not pretty, seen from the vantage point of gaining potential awareness, the chick is cracking through its eggshell and is about to learn how to walk around in a new world. While clearly this can happen more than once in a lifetime, here is one example of what this phase of our lives can look like.

The Movement from Acquired (Man/Woman) into Potential (Male/Female) Awareness

Paul was recovering from a vicious, drawn-out, and bitter divorce. After more than a few losing battles, he took the road of "letting her have it all" because he decided his sanity was worth more than his stuff or his ego. Years into the battle, things got so crazy his son sued his mother for stealing his college funds and won the suit. During a period of separation, Paul began to explore his masculine potential by doing things he had never done for himself. He moved into an apartment, learned to cook, changed the structure of his business, and became closer to his children in the process. Once the financial issues were settled, he began to date and drew up plans to build his dream home.

Viewed from the other side of this coin, Paul's former wife, Shelly, was also shedding her acquired awareness and exploring her feminine potential. She was utterly fed up with his preoccupation with his work and over the years became bored with their lifestyle. While he traveled, she stayed home. While he met all kinds of interesting people, she ate alone. She was the one who arranged family holidays, maintained the house, took care of the kids. After putting aside her own interests for nearly twenty years, she had had enough. Needless to say, sex was hardly something to look forward to, and there were many times she thought about what it would be like to be with someone else.

Once the divorce battles were through, she withdrew from financial entanglements and started to develop her career skills. She made new friends, took up golf, finished her degree, and started exploring her options as a single woman. Though her transitions were sometimes lonely and her future unknown, her renewed sense of independence made it all worthwhile.

Although this shift from acquired to potential awareness may take many years, eventually the fights and hopelessness subside and are replaced with new questions. What would I really like to be doing? What do I desire sexually? What do I want in a relationship? These are the kinds of questions we hear when our new female and male potential awareness is taking shape beyond the mold of acquired awareness.

Now, instead of merely being a man pursuing all kinds of ideas, dropping seeds, and having unconscious sex, he starts to care for the consequences of his conceptions. As his potential male awareness enters his consciousness, he looks for greater meaning in what he is doing. His battles mellow, and he begins to want more emotionally satisfying sexual experiences. For the woman stepping into her female potential, instead of being a receptacle carrying the seeds of others, she becomes more aware of the actions she must take to bring her receptivity to fruition. Through the exploration of being fully female, her eggs become more than overwhelming, unhatched possibilities. They start manifesting into clear, conscious conceptions. Sexually, she wants to expand out of her box and is curious to try new things.

The Movement Toward Evolutionary Awareness
Developing Masculine and Feminine Balanced Principles

As potential awareness shifts into evolutionary awareness, there will be alternating emotional outbursts and moodiness mixed with periods of peacefulness and calm. The transition into evolutionary awareness, which may take a lifetime to sustain, can be recognized by less tension, fewer struggles, and more enduring cycles of clarity, vitality, and contentment. In the beginning, the states in which our awareness is crystal clear seem to appear by accident. During peak moments, such as being present at a birth or death, or having a high-level orgasm, our awareness opens into bursts of receptive spontaneity.

During the exploration of our female and male potentials, we begin to consider the effects of our actions more carefully, and we become more sensitive to the needs of others. Eventually, as we gain glimpses of evolutionary awareness, battles for control and power are replaced by taking great pleasure when surprising abilities come out in ourselves and others. As men become more intuitive and women act more instinctively, we rely on each other with greater appreciation of our differences. These are signs of more harmonious masculine and feminine balance. As we experience more moments of evolutionary awareness, we have fewer stressful reactions, we are less attached to possessions, and life has much more humor. Things that seemed catastrophic, unattainable, or completely unchangeable become interesting challenges. Fixed roles and positions we once fought and suffered over are more flexible, and new forms of relationship are plausible. Rather than having to rely on making drastic external changes, we can often completely change the course of situations by shifting our internal attitudes. As we explore the potentials of our gender, former limitations evolve into assets. We will explore this in greater detail in later chapters regarding male-female instinctual differences.

While we are developing more balanced feminine and masculine principles of awareness, everything about sex changes significantly too. Our striving for positions of dominance or equality vanishes as jealousy fades away, pleasure comes more easily, and our sexual differences become the source of our attraction. When we are making love within the dynamic harmony of balanced feminine and masculine principles, we take all our female and male potential awareness with us. In fact, the more fully feminine and masculine we become, the more we are able to express intense passion. We neither crave nor avoid opportunities, and we start to gain tremendous energy from our sexual encounters. As expectations, possessiveness, and selfishness lose their appeal, we become far more creative lovers.

Entering evolutionary awareness is the place in human evolution that Quodoushka calls moving from the consciousness of karma into dharma. During the stages of karmic consciousness, we evolve more slowly and must learn over and over again by making countless mistakes. Within the consciousness of dharma perception, instead of needing to learn by making repeated mistakes, we learn faster through opportunities. For example, when we lose a job or a lover that causes a major piece of our identity to collapse, we see the situation as an opportunity to evolve.

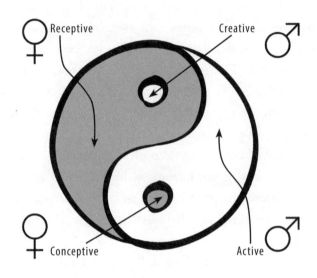

Fig. 4.5. Feminine-Masculine Principles/Energy Differences

THE FEMININE PRINCIPLE: RECEPTIVE—CREATIVE—CONCEPTIVE

Receptive means we must first be open enough to conceive, imagine, or envision something. Being conceptive means we allow the time it takes for an idea, a child, or a concept to grow internally. Creative means we remain open to different options and then take only the necessary and proper actions. Staying creative in our actions is the yang (action) within the yin (receptive).

The difference between discovering our female potential and activating a fully balanced feminine principle is great. Within female potential awareness, it means you are only receptive and not creative. In potential awareness, you start something, but then lose patience. It is as if, while you were waiting for plants to grow, you went out in the middle of the night, pulled them up a few inches, and then wondered why they all died the next morning. Sexually, it means you are open in the beginning, but when something doesn't go your way, you react negatively. You may communicate more honestly, but when your partner doesn't respond the way you want, you withdraw and wonder what's wrong.

Keep in mind, there is no shortcutting the time it takes to explore and test what works in our potential female awareness. During the stage of evolutionary awareness, developing our balanced feminine principle requires the wisdom and patience we gain only from experiencing things for ourselves. When we become fully balanced in what is called destiny or creational awareness, the craving for security and control is replaced with spontaneous intuition. We gain the ability to make proper discernments and we act with minimum effort and maximum efficiency. What does this look like sexually? Never twice the same. Each and every intimate encounter fluidly unfolds into an entirely unique experience. Although we will have intense orgasms more often, we know how to turn ordinary moments into extraordinary ones.

THE MASCULINE PRINCIPLE: ACTIVE—CREATIVE—CONCEPTIVE

When you are operating within the masculine principle, you start with an action and then stay creatively committed and connected to what you started. You remain open and flexible through the entire process in order to take care of whatever comes as a result of your actions. If you are operating in potential of male awareness, you are still exploring the outcomes and results of your actions. For example, when you are in the middle of doing something, you push through without noticing something is off. Then, when it turns out badly, you look to others to explain what went wrong. Sexually, you might be in the midst of having intercourse, but you do not realize your partner isn't that into it. If you do sense something off, you keep quiet. Afterward, you fail to see when you "checked out" and become disappointed because it wasn't a great time. You were more focused on the potential of what you were trying to make happen than noticing what was actually going on.

When we operate in the balanced masculine principle of awareness, it's quite a different experience. Let's say the same events took place, and you noticed you didn't have the greatest time making love. Within the masculine principle of awareness, even if you missed the initial moment when you disconnected from your lover, you recover quickly and talk about it. Rather than ignoring or covering up a "mistake," you might say, "I noticed there was a moment when I got distracted by thoughts of work. Did you feel when that happened?" Or perhaps you dressed sexy and tried to initiate sex, but your partner was too busy to notice. Instead of turning away and pouting, you decide to cook the evening's meal while seductively removing your new attire. In this manner, by staying creative in the flow of spontaneous action, a potentially disturbing situation turns into an opportunity for even more intimacy.

The balanced masculine principle of awareness means you take an action, stay flexible and responsive, and then take care of what happens as a result. Staying in a conceptive state of mind in our actions is the yin principle within the yang. Again, it is important to remember that masculine and feminine principles are not limited to gender; we are all made from the mixture of feminine and masculine energies.

Creational (or Destiny) Awareness

When we go from acquired to potential into evolutionary awareness, we go from being a woman to being fully female. As we evolve, we are able to hold more balanced feminine principles of awareness. Likewise, we evolve from being a man to being fully male—until we are able to live within balanced masculine principles of awareness. Creational awareness is the point in our maturation where we are able to embody the feminine receptive and masculine active principles of awareness that take us beyond gender and step us into our magical, mysterious character as fully balanced humans. Our magical, mysterious character is the part of us that is aware of our destiny to live according to the spontaneous wisdom of our Natural Self. The ultimate purpose of Quodoushka is to duplicate the sacred marriage of feminine and masculine creational energies called WahKahn and SsKwan inside us. It is our destiny to discover and become fully receptive-creative and active-conceptive human beings.

◎ Sexual Flowering Tree Ceremony
Gaining Awareness in Harmony with Nature

In this ceremony you are asked to find a tree in a safe, quiet place and take the time to engage in personal reflections. You will be exploring underlying issues that cause imbalances in your choreography and that block you from experiencing your feminine and masculine potential.

You will need to find a comfortable place with a tree you can sit against, where you can be alone to ask yourself the questions that follow. Answer each one and contemplate your responses. Take your time and savor your reflections, roll them around in your mind until the sweetness of understanding fills your awareness. You may wish to write your thoughts in a journal.

When the following "enemies" of doubt, insecurity, fear, repression, guilt, blame, and shame enter our awareness, they disrupt our natural equilibrium, and they keep us trapped in the limitations of acquired awareness. Answering these questions with honesty brings us into masculine/feminine potential awareness.

What You Will Need: A tree in a quiet, secluded place. A journal and pen. A pinch of tobacco, or a natural herb. You will also need to have a copy of the questions you are going to ask. It is always a good idea to tell a friend where you will be. This ceremony can take half an hour, or much longer. That's up to you.

To Begin: Once you find a suitable tree, walk around it three times in a clockwise direction. This is to create a sense of specialness and help bring you into a reflective mood. Trees and plants sit in the South of the wheels and thus help us balance our emotions.

What To Do: Sit with your back toward or against the tree facing each direction. For instance, when you are asking the South questions, your back will be against the tree and you will be looking out toward the south.

South: Emotional Sexual Doubts

Doubts block us from expressing our sexual needs and desires. Constantly doubting whether we are attractive or desirable enough, or whether we deserve pleasure, we seek ways to fit in with anyone who will support us. Whenever we question whether we are wanted, we are craving emotional approval, trying to make up for something we think we lack.

- How and when do I doubt myself and hold back sexually because I am afraid of being rejected?
- How do I use my sexuality in manipulative ways to be liked or loved?
- How do I use sexuality to stay in control?

North: Mental Sexual Insecurity

This is where we operate from the acquired awareness that does not serve us. Because we lack knowledge that works, we pursue credentials and place ourselves in relationships and situations that compromise our principles and suppress our natural feelings. Insecurity compels us to seek constant recognition from others. This is what leads us to conform to other people's rules and laws instead of discovering our own.

- What do I feel most insecure about in my sexual life?
- What or who do I depend on to make me feel sexually attractive?
- How and when do I hold back sexually when I am not recognized?

West: Physical Sexual Fears

The biggest fears we have are loneliness, old age, sickness, and death. When we try to find physical security based on these fears, we depend on relationships or our economic world to find safety just so we can belong. When we neglect our health, we add fuel to these fears, and we cannot access our inner resources.

- What are my greatest sexual fears?
- How am I not taking responsibility for my physical health?
- How do I use my lack of energy to avoid intimate connection?

East: Spiritual Sexual Repression

In our need to be spiritually accepted or "saved," we join groups and religions that make us feel connected to something larger than ourselves. We step into illusions by accepting opinions that repress our true nature, weaken our spiritual determination, and limit our ability to express sexual passion.

- What interferes with my free will to be more sexual?
- What makes me feel restless, unfulfilled, or sexually hopeless?
- Which of my words, feelings, or actions keep me from expressing sexual pleasure?

Center: Sexual Guilt, Blame, and Shame

When we look for our identity outside ourselves, needing to be seen as a perfect parent, husband, wife, or lover, we create rigid morals and ethics. When the morals and ethics we use to guide our sexual choices are created from guilt, blame, or shame of our Natural Self, we block access to our receptivity and creativity. We lose proper balance and alignment, and we cannot catalyze with passion and lust for life.

- Is there anything about my sexual life that I feel guilty or ashamed about?
- What part of my sexual identity must I keep hidden?
- How am I blaming others for sabotaging my sexual opportunities?

To complete the ceremony: After you have answered the questions, take some time to write a vow or a personal resolve to do something differently in each direction.

It is always good to leave a place looking better than when you arrived, so make sure you take away any trace of your having been there. It is also customary during this ceremony to leave a small token of thanks as a way of expressing appreciation for the opportunity to do the ceremony in a beautiful place. This can be a strand of hair, or more traditionally, you can leave a pinch of tobacco or a natural herb by the tree.

5

THE LIGHT AND DARK
ARROWS OF SEX

*When you begin to investigate, you notice, for one thing,
that whenever there is pain of any kind—the pain of
aggression, grieving, loss, irritation, resentment, jealousy,
indigestion, physical pain—if you really look into that,
you can find out for yourself that behind the pain there
is always something we are attached to. There is always
something we're holding on to.*

PEMA CHODRUN

SEVEN DARK ARROWS

Something happens that causes you to tighten. The habit of shooting dark
arrows begins with an impulse, an almost unnoticeable hook that triggers
an urge to close down. Your partner rejects a kiss. One minute her face is
open and relaxed, the next minute her jaw tenses. Her eyes roll upward,
and you get the cold shoulder. What's happening? You find yourself resisting your lover's touch. For some reason, you pull back with a tight "No."
When automatic reactions like these run you, then deeply pleasurable,
passionate sex becomes rare and unlikely.

It can happen a hundred times a day. Your body has a familiar tension. Once you start to notice this tendency, you feel it has been going on forever. Quodoushka calls it the dark arrow of attachment. It is said that we walk around with a quiver of twenty-one arrows that are the possible ways we can respond to any situation. When something provokes us to tighten, we reach for a dark arrow and get hooked so fast it seems like there's no choice at all. Before we know it, a flood of negativity is off and running.

Most of the time we don't even remember what set off the involuntary tightening, and we usually don't even realize we are tense. Then we react by trying to get rid of the feeling of unease. This is when you know you are wedged in by a dark arrow of attachment.

Once we grab this dark arrow, we're hooked. In less than a millisecond we close down, stirring the internal nest of doubt, contempt, or irritation that leads to poisonous words and actions. Remember movies where archers shoot swarms of arrows so thick they darken the sky? That's how it feels. Even if you want to stop, you don't. You can't stop because you are attached to the well-known destructive pattern.

Even though we know that spewing dark arrows from our mouths and minds is only going to make things worse, we can't pull them back. But the idea is not to get rid of them. In fact, hating our own negativity simply redirects the arrows and makes it harder to dig ourselves out of the hole. The only way to change course is by recognizing the initial tightening and learning to see how it quickly turns into dependencies, judgments, comparisons, and expectations.

Sometimes you catch yourself right away; other times it's only after the pit is dark and deep. It doesn't matter when you catch the habit. What matters is that you press the Pause button as soon as you can and pick up the first light arrow of awareness.

How Dark Arrows Work:
The Anatomy of Arguments

Your lover says something critical in the morning. You try to brush it off and move on with your day, but you can't let it go. You barely notice you are distant or that your habitual reactions are brewing, and even if you do, you don't care. You either grumble inside with resentment, repeating the offense, or you lash out in automatic defiance.

Within every attachment there is something we want. It can be as simple as wanting an apology after the insult. Although you may actually want connection, you cannot ask. So when the insult hits, you automatically press your feelings down, until eventually they come out sideways. This is how we turn an attachment into a dependency. As the difficulty worsens, it grows from something we want into something we need.

When we get trapped inside the routine of our dependencies, we get locked into positions of conflicting needs. Things as petty as how the dishes get cleaned, leaving socks on the floor, having too many lights on, or arguing about who had the last orgasm become fuel for more irritation. Whenever we shoot an arrow of dependency, we need the other to maintain his or her position, even if it's destructive. Then we make things worse with the third dark arrow of judgment.

Judgment extends the tension into separation. This is the point of arguments where the original offense is forgotten and what started as a spat careens into a full-fledged battle. You say to yourself, "I can't stand this." By now the all-too-familiar roles are hardened into place. Whether you take the stance of the persecutor, victim, or rescuer, judgment insists your position is right and the other is not.

Next, the dark arrow of comparison rears its head. You start bringing in past episodes, or getting others to take your side. As we stretch this out for hours or days, we then begin to hurl dark arrows of expectation— complaints like, "Why are you always so critical?" or "Why do you always walk away?" All these emotions are actually habitual reactions from the past. After a while, a kind of numbness sets in with the feeling, "This will never end" or "There is no way out." Expectations are also demands that in one way or another say, "You should do what I want." As the tension mounts and separation widens, with the dark arrows flying in full force, we try our best tactics to gain control. It's maddening, but it's not over yet.

The Mask of Self-Pity

This bundle of negativity coalesces into what is called the needy, wounded, abandoned child syndrome. The process is called the Circle of Foxes because we are setting ourselves up to chase our tails, and we do this over and over again. The same arguments keep erupting no matter how many discussions we have. The rejections, the sulking, and the childish demands lie in wait for the trigger to be pulled. The dark arrows compound into an indulgent, narcissistic sense of entitlement called the Mask of Self-Pity. The needy, wounded, and abandoned child wants approval, recognition, security, and acceptance. Surely we have outgrown these needs, but in reality we have only smoothed over habits.

The Mask of Self-Importance

This is when the next dark arrows kick in. We don't like appearing needy, and we don't like admitting we can't control our emotional outbursts. So we cover our self-pity with yet another dark arrow: the clever Mask of Self-Importance. Every time we are arrogant or jealous, or act like a self-righteous martyr, we are hiding behind the mask of self-importance. Even when get what we want, there is no escape. We only activate more attachments and then have to protect what we've got. Underneath all these masks we are still restless, tight, and uneasy. We feel defeated by the tyrants of life—the relationship, the job, or the government—and believe that they are somehow responsible for our predicament. Yet we carry on pretending we are fine—that is, until something else happens. It's a devastating syndrome.

THE SEVEN LIGHT ARROWS

Although these patterns may feel like they are hardwired into our brains and bodies, and just about anything can yank our chain on a bad day, we are not wired to keep picking up dark arrows forever. It is entirely possible to refrain from our habitual urges and do something different.

Since it is easier to observe in milder situations, let's rewind the scenario. Something happens. An insult comes flying at you in the morning. You notice you're tightening, and you feel yourself about to react, but instead of trying to get unhooked, you lean *into* the feeling of tension. In this instant you are picking up the first light arrow of awareness. As soon as you divert your attention to notice your own tension, it takes your finger off the trigger. It is a deliberate choice that feels like, "Hmm, I'm feeling a bit tense. Interesting." Pressing the Pause button of awareness brings you into the present moment. At this point, you don't have to do anything except notice yourself.

Congratulations, you have just opened the door for the rest of the light arrows to come rushing in. Self-awareness leads to self-appreciation and self-acceptance. These are the self-worth arrows. They give you breathing space to appreciate, for one thing, that you did not slip into another reaction. They give you room to accept the entire situation. You start to realize that what was said has nothing to do with you. It feels like a Tai Chi move, in which, instead of putting your face in front of a fist, you take a slight step to the side and watch the fist whiz past. If we let go of the urge to withdraw, fix, defend, or attack, we can simply appreciate the situation for what it is. What's happening is neutral; what matters is how we respond.

On a good day like this, when we manage to avoid the small calamities that might turn into disasters, watching what is happening becomes amusing and even pleasurable. Catching ourselves in the act and averting discord sets off a new trajectory of light arrows. If we can allow self-pleasure, even in the face of discord, especially if we can open ourselves sexually, we gain insights into the heart of our lover's desires, and we attract the arrow of self-love. These are the times when we drop the fight, spontaneously decide to make love, and gain the magical gifts of high-level orgasms.

Self-Actualization

When we can reach into our quiver of possibilities and no longer habitually grab for dark arrows, it is called entering Warrior's Freedom. As we learn to respond to each situation according to the nuances of present conditions, we discover the arrow of self-actualization. It does not mean you will instantly live happily ever after by manifesting the woman, the house, or the man of your dreams. With this light arrow, relationships, sex, intimacy, worldly skills, and many things that once seemed out of reach start to happen more easily.

When things start going our way however, we feel elated and have a tendency to think we have arrived. Gaining the ability to actualize with ease inevitably produces a breeze of confidence along with smug feelings of invincibility. This is when the light arrow of self-awareness is needed most. As is said in Sun Tsu's *The Art of War,* defeat is often close at hand at the moment of victory; or, as others say, "Pride cometh before the fall." Here too, at the climax of great sex, after accomplishing fantastic things, we are most vulnerable to defeat. Whenever we begin to actualize our dreams and desires with greater ease, it is time for great caution because new attachments are close at hand.

What we are truly actualizing is not wealth, nor great sex; it's a relaxed, unattached awareness. Let's say some long-hoped-for dream comes true and you finally meet the man or woman of your dreams. Self-actualization keeps you on the precipice of awareness where you realize these precious gifts require great care and focus to sustain.

Impeccability

Entering Warrior's Freedom, we pick up the light arrow of impeccability. We finally listen less to the grasping ambitions of our lower self and can hear the calling of our higher self to evolve. It is different than trying to be perfect. Acting with impeccability means we have done the absolute best we can do. An Olympic champion can have an impeccable loss as long as he or she has completely applied himself or herself on a given day.

As we begin to shoot light arrows into the world, it's not that loss or conflicts disappear or that we remain permanently calm. What changes is that we see our limitations and our gifts more clearly. Being impeccable is a matter of continual refinement as we look for how we can truly be of service to others. As we drop grudges and grievances about the way things are, we cultivate compassion for our own and other people's flaws. Being an impeccable warrior also means to take responsibility and stand accountable for both our transgressions and our shining.

The Seven Rainbow Arrows

Rainbow Arrows are the spontaneous gifts of spiritual growth that often come to us in unpredictable and unexpected ways. *What* we do matters less then *how* we approach situations. Without exception, every time we choose a light arrow instead of a dark one, we initiate a stream of magnetic thoughts. Although we seldom see the arc of return or know the exact consequences of our actions, the more light arrows we send into the world, the more illumination, insights, trust, innocence, wisdom, and honest communication we will receive. With light arrows perched on our bow of self, spontaneous, spiritual, and deeply fulfilling sexual union becomes possible. Moreover, our relationships become rich, fertile ground for developing mutual support, in every way helping us actualize what we were born to do. The seventh Rainbow Arrow brings the gifts of abundance, prosperity, and the true wealth of our soul's contentment.

THE LIGHT AND DARK ARROWS

The Seven Dark Arrows	The Seven Light Arrows	The Seven Rainbow Arrows
Circle of Foxes Our Karma Circle at the Effect of our Shideh (Lower Self)	Dance of the Coyote Our Dharma Circle at Cause, Listening to our Hokkshideh (Higher Self)	Walk of the Wolf Transformation Circle the Gifts of Co-Empowerment
Attachments	Self-Awareness	Illumination
Dependencies	Self-Acceptance	Introspection
Judgments	Self-Appreciation	Trust and Innocence

Comparisons	Self-Pleasure	Wisdom, Balance, and Alignment
Expectations	Self-Love	Heart-to-Heart Communication
Mask of Self-Pity	Impeccability	Male-Female Balance
Mask of Self-Importance	Self-Actualization	Abundance and Prosperity

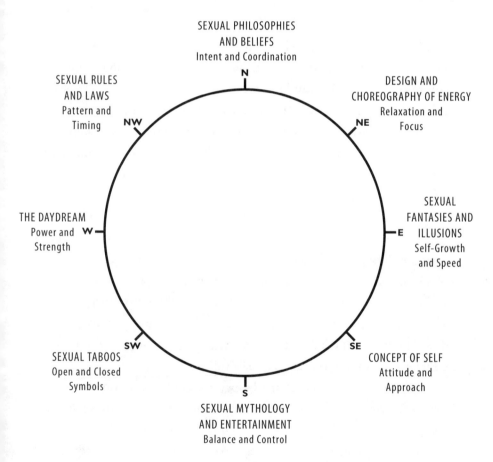

SEXUAL PHILOSOPHIES
AND BELIEFS
Intent and Coordination
N

SEXUAL RULES
AND LAWS
Pattern and
Timing   NW

DESIGN AND
CHOREOGRAPHY OF ENERGY
Relaxation and
NE   Focus

THE DAYDREAM
Power and   W
Strength

SEXUAL
FANTASIES AND
E   ILLUSIONS
Self-Growth
and Speed

SW

SE

SEXUAL TABOOS
Open and Closed
Symbols

CONCEPT OF SELF
Attitude and
Approach

S
SEXUAL MYTHOLOGY
AND ENTERTAINMENT
Balance and Control

Fig. 5.1. The Star Maiden's Circle

THE SEXUAL STAR MAIDENS CIRCLE

Legend has it that this wheel is derived from observations made by the Star Maidens or the sisters of the Pleiades, who, it is said, upon watching human folly from a distant star created the wheel to describe the full gamut of earthly human behavior. Regardless of whether we believe wise maidens from the stars had such a bird's-eye view, the wheel shows us how to mine the dark, often hidden sides of our sexual nature to turn unfortunate circumstances into the light.

South

Sexual Mythology and Entertainment

We all create myths about what happened to us as children. We tell stories about how we were given too little or too much affection, about how sex was kept out of sight and never talked about, or how our first sexual explorations were thwarted. If our parents cared for and loved us twenty-three hours a day, we remember that one missing hour. The attention we did not get from our mothers and fathers becomes the underlying theme of our myths, whereas the moments of genuine affection often stay locked away in our memory.

Woven into our dark stories are the ways we were scolded, felt smothered, abandoned, put down, and not loved. It's as if we store the wounds of our childhood in our bodies and turn them into "pain tapes" that burn holes in our psyches. The moment we feel let down or hurt, we revert to the tapes and play them out in our adult sex lives. If our partner threatens to leave, we react as if it were our father abandoning us all over again. We ask for permission, rebel, become moody, feel controlled and criticized, and try to get attention in the old painful ways.

You might ask, if our dark mythologies are so painful, why do we keep repeating them and entertaining ourselves with such unfulfilling dramas? The answer is that they are what we know. We tell our familiar tales of neglect or belittlement because we are used to them, and we are convinced that what happened to us is unchangeable. Our past gives us reasons to avoid intimacy, and we use our mythology to try to protect ourselves from further harm. The trouble is, repeating the old stories keeps new ones from happening. While certainly the tragic pain tapes of serious physical and emotional abuse are difficult to erase, it is possible to forgive even the gravest traumas and revise our stories. Along with picking up the arrow of awareness, reflecting on our dark mythology shines light into our victim stories and turns them around to our advantage.

If you could summarize the dark side of your childhood as if it were a movie, what would be the title?

Sheryl's Story:
"Good Girls Don't Do Things Like That"

It was a particular thing that happened when I was sixteen years old. My first boyfriend actually found out where I lived. I shared the name of the street, but not the house. When he figured out which house was mine, he knocked on my door, and said, "Hi," I was shocked. I couldn't believe he thought I was so attractive he would actually walk over to my house to find me. Our relationship got started one night when we went out for a date and we came back to my house. He was standing up against his car and we were hugging—stars were bursting out of our bodies. My mom saw me from the window in the den. When I came back inside, she said to me, "You know, you need to pay attention to what you are doing. Good girls don't do things like that."

That was a shock. It was confusing, and I suppose I felt a little guilty too. Something was not right, but I didn't know exactly what it was. I figured it must have been the sexual spark-flying moment when your bodies touch and the lightning stream of pleasure goes through your body. The message my sixteen-year-old brain got was, "I've got to make sure that if I do this again, no one else is going to see me, especially my mother." But it felt great, and I didn't want to give it up. From then on I had to be careful about how I showed passion. I didn't know it back then, but I was setting up a story I used many times as an adult.

Whether the bruises our Natural Self takes on are mild or much more traumatic, stories like these lay the groundwork for how we act later on as adults. Are we shy about showing affection? Are we hesitant to initiate sexual play? Are we cautious, restrained, or afraid of rejection? Or are we overly bold and insensitive?

REWRITING YOUR STORY:
"GOOD GIRLS FEEL GOOD"

Once you have named your dark story, practice rewriting your history, casting yourself as the hero or heroine. To find the light title of your movie, try to recall small victories and instances of courage you experienced as a child. Look for times you triumphed and were loved. It's important to name your dark title first, because it carries the nuances and trigger words of negative emotions you keep playing out. Other dark titles might be, "Tough Guy Gets Going," "Second Place Joe," or "Not Smart Enough." You know you have found your dark movie title when saying it conjures up the doubts, fears, and insecurities you felt as a kid. The light title should instill hope, confidence, and inspiration. It can be used as a mantra to loosen the grip of blame, shame, or guilt and helps you view what is happening from a different angle.

Turning around negative stories can dramatically change the course of your relationships. "Not Smart Enough" could become "My Brilliance Is Me." For Sheryl, "Good Girls Don't Do Things Like That" turned into "Good Girls Feel Good." This powerful inner message of self-acceptance and self-worth comes from whittling away old ingrained emotions and creating experiences where "It's okay to feel good."

Here is what is interesting about pain-tape stories. Hidden inside the hurts, wounds, and confusions we experienced as young boys or girls are also the gems of victory. While we may not be able to change the "facts" of what happened to us, instead of unconsciously replaying and rebelling against our story, we can always change our attitude about what happened. The reality is that our parents, siblings, or anyone who inflicted harm was acting out of ignorance, and they were doing the best they could at the time.

Our early curiosities and fantastic explorations into the world of sexual feelings are often obstructed by someone telling us we were bad or wrong. The question is, which messages will we weave into our lives and carry to our graves? Notice in Sheryl's story there is also the part where the heroine says, "It felt great, and I didn't want to give it up." Embedded within everything that happens are also the seeds of our strength and determination to grow and learn. If you could turn around your dark story, what would be the title of your light movie?

Southwest
Sexual Taboos: Open and Closed Symbols

Any object, thing, person, or event that enters our consciousness is called a Symbol of the Dream, because we ascribe meaning to whatever we encounter within our waking or sleeping dreams. An open symbol is something we interpret positively, and a closed symbol is something we may be curious about, but have not tried.

Our sex lives are typically filled with open and closed symbols. We might be curious about what it would be like to have sex with someone of the same sex but will not go near the taboo. We like kissing but may shy away from anal sex. We may be fascinated by the darker sides of sex but have never let ourselves be blindfolded. You might have a closed symbol about visiting a swingers' club, viewing the scene as tawdry and crude. Nonetheless, swingers' clubs keep coming up on your radar screen to pique your interest. What would it be like to walk around in a place where everyone is openly and obviously interested in sex?

The Swingers' Club

I had heard about them for years, but every time the subject came up, I shut the door, thinking that it was horribly wrong. It seemed like the more I tried not thinking about them, the more swingers' clubs came up in conversations. It seemed like everyone was talking about them, and nearly everyone had been to one except me. Finally, my curiosity got the best of me, so I decided to go with a friend, just to have a look.

Sure enough, when we got past the entrance and came into the dimly lit club, it looked like I expected, with red leather chairs, red carpet, and red velvet curtains covering the doors. I saw people walking toward side rooms and back doors. I was fascinated, but I didn't dare go to see what they were doing. I almost wanted to dash out the door but decided to stay and have a drink with my friend. All the TV shows I had seen were nothing quite like being there. It felt like every person who walked by, both women and men, gave me the once-over. I had to go to the bathroom, but there was no way I was going to venture in there by myself, so I just stayed at the bar. I know lots of people are into this sort of thing, but to me it was overwhelming. Just when I was thinking these things, a lady came and sat next to me. We actually had a great conversation because it turned out she was nervous about being there too. My friend went off into one of those back rooms as we watched people from the bar. We joked about what my friend was probably doing. It was the best casual encounter I have ever had, and I can't believe it happened that night.

I haven't been back to a swingers' club since then. It made me realize that I prefer an intimate, cozy night with someone I know. When I find that person, maybe we will go explore a club like that together. In fact, I think it could be a lot of fun now that it's not so terrifying.

DON

When we have a strong charge about something we deem taboo, it costs us a great deal of energy to keep it locked away and usually consumes more energy than what it would take to discover something about it. When taboos are too tightly shunned, they can become perverted and destructive. Sometimes, what is really behind a closed symbol that we refuse to look at is a fear that we may actually like what's behind the door. Of course, there are plenty of things that may be too much, like walking naked to your mailbox or having sex while skydiving. At the same time, there may be things you have always wanted to do, but just never found the nerve.

Flipping Fear into Passion: Oral Sex

I don't know why, but I was never into oral sex. Getting it was not a problem at all, but for some reason I did not want to give oral sex to my partner. It got to be a real issue, because I knew my girlfriend wanted it, but when she would ask, I just could not do it. I thought I would hurt her feelings if I said I didn't enjoy it all that much.

Finally one day I decided I had to talk about the way I felt. I told her I thought she was beautiful, and that I had no idea what turned me off, or why I avoided giving to her in that way. It was such a relief to talk, and her reaction totally surprised me. She took it on as a kind of project and suggested we watch a couple of videos with lots of oral sex. I had never thought of watching porno movies to improve my sex life, but I was open to anything that would work. Despite my fears, I really did want to give her pleasure.

I think it was seeing two women licking and kissing each other's vaginas that did the trick. I started to get a hard-on while we were watching it. My girlfriend took my head and brought it toward her open thighs. She asked me just to look at first, and had me gaze and appreciate her beautiful vagina. But that was it. We didn't do anything else at first. We did this several more times, each time getting a little closer, and a little more turned on. Once, she had me bathe and pat her dry. I guess I was so turned on by her patience with me that I finally really wanted to taste and caress her with my mouth. Since that time, I have come to appreciate how lovely she is, and it has become one of my favorite ways of bringing her to orgasm. I don't know what I was so afraid of, but I am glad we took the time to get past my fears.

STEPHAN

Opening a closed symbol does not have to be a reckless leap into the unknown. At times it is better to take small, careful steps toward facing our closed symbols. It is always important to be safe, and there is never a good reason to put yourself in any kind of danger. There are times, however, when directly facing your biggest fears and taking a spontaneous leap into something unknown helps you break through illusionary barriers. Remember heart-pounding moments like walking across the dance floor hoping someone would say yes? Or when you made love the very first time? Going into the unknown from time to time creates some of the most exhilarating and memorable experiences of our lives.

The dark side of opening closed symbols is using sex as a thrill factory by trying to quench our thirst for instant gratification and constantly craving new exploits. Although variety and adventure can be interesting sources of pleasure, they can also quickly lose their appeal. We can get addicted to the dopamine rush of novelty. The key to successfully bringing new experiences into your sex life is to use them sparingly, as a spice rather than as a main course. If you notice you are stuck in a lull, then it may be a good time to do something you have never done. Things like going to a sex shop and picking up an anal vibrator, having sex in an elevator, or doing it in the car may work for some. In case these don't do it for you, try simply initiating sex out of the blue if you usually don't. There is tremendous potential for passion, pleasure, and knowledge behind any closed symbol we open with care.

West

The Daydream

The West of the wheel is the place of death, change, transformation, and renewal. It is the part of our lives where we put things off into the future as if we will live forever. Buddhists say that the opportunity to be born into a human body can be likened to a turtle swimming in the ocean. On the surface, floating somewhere in the vast sea, is an inner tube. The chances of being born through a physical womb are like the odds of the turtle reaching the surface and popping its head through the middle of the ring.

The dark side of the daydream is when we coast lazily through life, forgetting the preciousness of our body and its true needs. We get caught in routines and schedules and avoid occasions for deep sexual intimacy. The French call an orgasm a *petite mort,* or little death. Opening ourselves sexually and surrendering into orgasm is a deep letting-go in which we come face to face with our own mortality and feel the impermanence of life.

In shamanic teachings, it is said we must wake up from the daydream by learning to make death an ally. This means waking from our sleepiness with an awareness that we can die at any moment. If you have ever had a near-death experience in which you have seen scenarios of your life flashing by, you have had a glimpse of how death can jolt you into cherishing life. When we treat our sexual unions as opportunities to celebrate the beauty of being alive, then all the insecurities we have about our physical bodies, including how we look, how much we weigh, or whether we can perform can be put in proper perspective.

Karen's Story: The Change of Life

When I was young I was pretty thin, and my weight could go up and down. Then I reached a point where it seemed to go up and up, and it was practically impossible to take off. I know why they call it the "change of life" because a lot of things have changed. I became more self-conscious about my body. Issues I had as a girl, ones I thought I had resolved, came rushing back with a vengeance. On the one hand, I was facing getting older; at the same time, teenage emotions were swarming inside like angry bees.

When I first went through menopause, there were so many things unknown to me. Inside I was still young, and sometimes I wanted to have sex in a New York minute. But I became wary to even approach a man because I didn't look the way I felt inside. That part of me, that confidence, was on the back burner because I didn't want to face any kind of rejection. I felt deflated and resigned. I had to go through many transitions to get back that sexy part of myself. It was difficult.

Gradually, something began to change. As I reflected deep inside myself, I had to face my inner fears and monsters. I had to face the fact that my body was changing, and I had to find the determination to change the way I ate, the way I exercised, and the way I rested. I started to have a new sense of care about my body. During this time I realized that my bottled-up emotions were causing me to feel bloated and stuck. At one point, when I got honest about resentments, confronted them, and then let these emotions go, I actually started my period again for several months. It was an amazing feeling, as if a river had burst through a dam.

Since that time, I have carefully tended to both my emotions and my lifestyle. I know having negative feelings about my body shuts down my sexual desires. I may not be able to turn back the clock, but I am determined to let my inner nymph, that young part of myself, come out to play more. Feeling sexy is a big part of who I am, and there's no way I am going to give that up. Through all the changes, I am realizing that what I want sexually now is different from what it used to be. In a way, I am wiser, and perhaps more mellow about sex, but I can see a light at the end of the tunnel. It is kind of exciting. One thing I can say is that when I feel even slightly horny now, I do something about it. I make sure I appreciate the sexy feelings I do have, and I initiate connections whenever I can. Reducing my insecurities and resentments has made facing the unknown changes of life into a challenging yet remarkable adventure.

Northwest
Sexual Rules and Laws

Many of the rules and laws we have surrounding sexuality allow us to respect each other's privacy and keep us from using our sexual energy in harmful ways. Protecting the sanctity of children and maintaining clear rules around mutual consent are certainly necessary and beneficial laws. Many social rules, however, keep us from expressing our natural sexual feelings and corner us into overly constricting boxes. It's not that someone builds these rules for us; it's more that our entire conditioning forms an invisible container where we feel safe inside. The work of deciding which rules and laws support the awakening of our Natural Self is what Quodoushka calls remembering our Sacred Image.

Climbing Out of the Box

You have to be able to look at the box you are in and clearly identify what it is made of. Can you push the boundaries of the box further? Is it flexible, or like steel? Which of your rules and laws are beneficial, and which ones are not? What happens if you want to initiate sex? What inner rules do you have inside that are keeping you too safe, and which ones are helping you grow and learn with pleasure?

Divorces, in one way or another, are an attempt to get out of the box we find ourselves in. At some point we grow out of the container we built. The question is, are you going to just build another one by jumping into another relationship box? During my first marriage there was a period when I was showing up to family holidays making excuses why my husband was not with me. I grew up internalizing rules that said when you are married, you do family things together, especially holidays. At some point I stopped ducking insults from in-laws and making excuses for my husband. I started to enjoy going by myself. When I went into my second marriage, I made some new rules, which have worked well for over fifteen years. One of them was that my husband and I are two separate human beings with our own individual interests. We love doing many things together, but there are certain things we do on our own. For me, this rule keeps our sanity and independence alive. There are so many things I wish to study and learn, and it is fantastic to have the freedom and support to do them. Widening my box of rules that work has not only given me room to explore who I am, it fills me with confidence and brings new energy to our sex life.

LAURA

North
Sexual Philosophies and Beliefs

Our sex lives are riddled with beliefs that limit opportunities for intimate connection. Sexual beliefs are often rooted in the stories of our youth. For example, the story of being abandoned by our fathers turns into perceptions that "Men always leave" or "Men are afraid of commitment," and the story of feeling overprotected by our mothers leads to the opinion that "Women are controlling." The trouble with these and other limiting beliefs, such as "There are no good men out there," or "Women reject me because . . . ," is that they wind up being self-fulfilling prophecies.

Since we tend to surround ourselves with people who think like we do, it's easy to get locked into perceiving only what we already believe. If we collect friends who are convinced that "Sexual passion always fades away" or that "Sex is too risky these days," we build up our assumptions and persuade each other they are true. One way to shift false thinking is to create friendships with people who have empowering, inspiring, and diverse ways of looking at things.

Another way is to explore having a sexual encounter by intentionally adopting another point of view. Try making love with the belief that "Women are mysterious" or that "Men are incredibly sensitive" and see what kinds of sexual experiences start to happen. Opening yourself to the idea that "Aging allows more subtle sensations of pleasure" will change the trajectory of your intimate experiences. Expressing these types of empowering beliefs is the most effective way to sustain interesting and passionate relationships.

William's Trip to Tibet: Beliefs between the Sheets

I came from a family of hard-working parents and was brought up to believe that success meant hard work. When I went to Tibet, we stayed in a large hut with several families living under one roof. They had so few material things that it was shocking to me at first. Everyone seemed to be quite busy and focused, yet there was something different about the way these people worked.

What impressed me most was the way they talked to each other in such an easygoing way. I couldn't understand what they were saying, but it was the tone of their voices and the way they would pause to look into each other's eyes that showed me something. For me, work meant you close off feelings and go off into your own world. They seemed to connect with a kind of intimacy no matter what they were doing.

I hadn't realized how much staying with them for that week affected me until I was with my wife in bed a week later. I remembered their melodic voices and started talking to my wife with the same tone while we were making love. Somehow, I took that easygoing focus to heart and began touching her body that way. She certainly liked it. To me it felt like a thousand beliefs I had about making love dropped away. I hadn't realized I approached sex like work, where things had to be methodical and hard. I couldn't believe such a simple shift, just relaxing a bit more and lightening up, could bring my wife such lovely pleasure.

Northeast
Design and Choreography of Energy

Ultimately, the small choices we make to either withhold or share intimacy are what constitute the reality of our sexual lives, and our decisions about how often to have sex are based upon what really matters to us. Are you too busy to give or receive pleasure? Do the children get in the way? Do you spend more time arguing than being intimate? Does food, shopping, talking, work, reading, watching TV, or just about anything crowd out time for sex? After it's all said and done, however important we say sex is, it's how we design our lives that exactly reflects our real priorities.

Recurring sexual frustrations, frequent dissatisfaction, loneliness, and exhaustion are signs you are out of alignment with the natural rhythms of desire. The universal excuse of being "too tired" for pleasure is always a result of a backward, chaotic choreography of energy. It's backward because rather than using sexual intimacy to *give* us energy for everything else we do, we keep it on the back shelf. Instead of letting sex take precedence over other things and doing whatever it takes to make it happen, we make the mistake of thinking it's too hard.

But creating a balanced lifestyle doesn't need to be difficult. Having a fulfilling sex life starts with clearing away clutter and deciding to bring your emotional, mental, physical, and spiritual choices into alignment with your true priorities. In other words, if you consider sexual intimacy vitally important, then you need to make choices and decisions in your daily life that support having more intimate sexual experiences.

Use the questions that follow to see what keeps you from making better sexual choices and decisions. Once you answer these questions, you will have a better idea how to have more fulfilling sexual experiences on a regular basis.

◎ A Personal Ceremony to Get Clear About Your Priorities
Creating an Agreement Between Self and Spirit

Emotional

How do my emotions keep me from enjoying sex and intimacy?

What can I do to calm my emotions?

Mental

How do I let stress and mental tension interfere with my sexual desires?

What activities calm my mind?

Physical

How do I let my physical health prevent me from having intimate sex?

What are three things I can commit to doing to improve my health?

Spiritual

How do my feelings of hopelessness or boredom limit my sexual expressions?

What do I enjoy doing most?

What can I commit to doing that will strengthen my spirit?

Sexual

What are my actual sexual needs?

How often would I like to have sex if I could?

What are three things I can do to have more sexual intimacy?

Considering theses questions and making new agreements with yourself and others gives you a better understanding of how important sexual intimacy is for you.

East
Sexual Fantasies and Illusions

Your secret fantasies tell you something about what your spirit needs to feel more expansive and alive. For example, if you need more passion and strength, you may see yourself being seduced by a dominant lover. If you desire more touch, you may dream of being sensuously aroused by several lovers. Imagining yourself as a sexual god or goddess reveling in carnal delight may mean you yearn for profound love. Used in this way, actualizing your fantasies feeds your spirit's hunger to experience pleasurable states of joyful union.

It can be fantastic to do something you have always wanted to do sexually, yet if you become obsessed with an image of a particular person or thrilling scene, your fantasies keep you lost in illusions. Wandering off and away from your partner, you get more turned on by appearances than by the warm body you are lying next to. You can also stray into the dark side when what used to be an exciting treat becomes the only thing that turns you on. Any time you fixate on fetishes or become too extreme, you will create situations that harm your spirit. The key to enjoying your fantasies in beneficial ways is to remember they rarely turn out the way you imagine. The secret to actualizing them is to stay open to how they might be played out, and look for opportunities to express your inner desires.

Kimberly on the Beach

I always had a fantasy about making love in nature, being completely out in the open, without a soul in sight, having the wind blowing over my whole body. For years, I used this fantasy to help me fall asleep, and as I imagined my lover making deep, passionate love to me, I always had a great orgasm before slipping into dreamtime.

I wasn't looking for this to happen, but when the opportunity came up, I went for it. A friend of mine invited me to a beach house he rented in Maine. One night we were walking on the shore listening to the waves break over our feet. We were reminiscing about good times when he suddenly grabbed me in his arms and started kissing me wildly. It all happened so naturally, curling onto the ground, sprawling our clothes onto the sand. The heat of our bodies made the chill of the night wind feel fantastic. We had sand and water all over our bodies, and I didn't care. I howled and moaned with sounds of love like I had never heard before. To this day, I think of that night as one of the most wonderful memories of my whole life.

Triple Fantasy in San Francisco

My fantasy was to be with two women. The way it finally happened was better than what I could have planned. I was staying in a resort near San Francisco, where two ladies I met at a wine-tasting party invited me back to their place. We built a fire, drank a bottle of vintage wine, and talked into the evening. It was getting late when one of the women came over to me and sat on my lap. She unzipped my trousers while her friend watched. I won't go into detail about everything that happened, but I will say that things got so hot I didn't know where my body began or ended and whose hands were doing what. I didn't know I could come so many times. The best part for me was watching them kissing passionately by the fire and stroking their bodies in sheer delight. Sometimes, a fantasy only happens once in a lifetime, but I certainly hope this one happens again.

PETER

Southeast
Concept of Self

Our attitude and approach to life, along with how we cast the light and dark arrows, establishes our concept of self. We continuously create our self concept by how we make our own great journey around the Star Maiden's Circle.

Our experiences in every direction determine the way we view the world. Rewriting your story and opening closed symbols keeps you out of the past and gives you more opportunities for magical sexual encounters. Adopting a more positive body image helps you get in touch with your need and desire for sexual expression. Expanding your box of rules starts by expressing sexual beliefs that work for you. Having a more balanced daily choreography gives you the energy to be creative and keeps you ready for sexy, spontaneous intimate adventures.

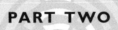

PART TWO

Language, Anatomy, and Orgasms

6

A Natural
Language for Sex

Language shapes the way we think, and the words we use carry messages about the way we feel. Imagine for a moment if a teenage girl was taught that her outer lips (if they were ever mentioned at all) are called "butterfly wings" as opposed to introducing them as her "labia majora." What if young men were taught they carried sacred jewels and precious seeds instead of testicles and semen?

When we are introduced to the world of sex and genitals, we hear words like *corpus spongiosm, urethra, scrotum, prostate, labium, cervix,* and *Fallopian tubes.* While most of these terms rarely find their way into our bedrooms, and they do serve a purpose, they are far from inspiring. The technical-sounding language we use to teach children and train doctors deliberately siphons out much of the beauty and rich complexities of sex. Derived mainly from Latin, our scientific jargon neutralizes the subject and keeps us at arm's length from feeling anything remotely sexual when we say them. The more common words we actually use, such as *vagina* or *penis,* while they do the job, are less than poetic at best, and they convey a sense of the dispassionate distance Westerners have toward sex.

Some of the recent terms established in the 1950s that are used to describe the various parts of our sexual anatomy come from the names of men who "discovered" or hypothesized their existence, such as the Bartholin glands or the Gräfenberg spot, now commonly known as the G-spot. Our sexual language often reveals the Western divide between our bodies and nature. While the Quodoushka names may not be as specific or precise, they are accurate, simple, and beautiful to say. Most of all, they convey an entirely different message about sex. They are inherently reverent, and as such teach us to regard ourselves, Mother Life, and our sexuality as sacred.

It is hard, for example, to say the word *tupuli* (pronounced ta-POOL'-lee) without having a slight smile on your lips by the time you finish saying it. It means a woman's vagina. *Tipili* (pronounced tee-PEEL'-lee), which invokes for us an image of an erect teepee, is the word for penis. Other names include Valley of Pleasure (perineum), Head of the Cobra (clitoris), Sacred Snake (penis), and Rear Cavern (anus). While it might be a stretch to think about a Harvard professor or a gynecologist saying, "We are going to examine the Head of the Cobra" or "check your Rear Cavern," the alternate names evoke something wonderful about sex. Using animals and images of nature to describe our sexual anatomy gives life to language and reflects inherently subtle, intricate, and sometimes poetic perceptions that are provocative and clear.

The language of Quodoushka also suggests the originators of these teachings, much in the same manner indigenous people insightfully observe animals, plants, and Earth's changes, were remarkably astute in their understanding of human sexuality. Whatever language we may use to describe our genitalia, it is refreshing and empowering to have words that portray our erogenous zones in a positive, endearing manner. Perhaps the specificity of Western terms, together with the more nature-based names of Quodoushka, can lay the foundation for becoming more aware and caring lovers. And perhaps if we bring these words into our most private conversations, or use them to teach our children, we can restore a sense of magic and mystery in our sexual lives.

MALE EROGENOUS ZONES
OF PLEASURE

In one respect, men are exactly like women: caressing or kissing their ears, lips, neck, inner thighs, or even behind their knees at the right moment can be totally erotic. While most men may not require extended foreplay to get aroused, many love it. One of the major differences between men and women's erogenous zones, however, is that males like attention to their tipilis sooner rather than later. The penis is by far the most sensitive erogenous zone in the male body.

The Penis Shaft:
Sacred Snake

According to his anatomy type, every man prefers certain kinds of pressure, speed, and types of movements along the shaft at various stages of their arousal. The timing of how these strokes are given is very important, and most men have a fairly specific way they like to be brought to climax.

While most men are happy to tell you faster, or slower, they probably won't articulate too clearly about what takes them to the highest states of

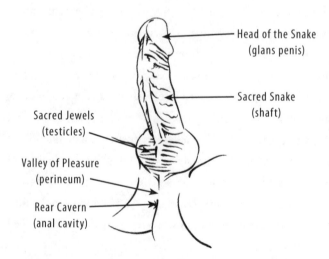

Fig. 6.1. The Tipili, or Sacred Snake, otherwise known as
the male sexual conceptive organ, or the penis

arousal. It's a mistake to assume that any strokes will do along the shaft. The fun part of becoming a more sensitive, caring lover is to discover what works best for him. Exploring a man's preferences, and learning to sense when he is about to ejaculate, as well as knowing just the kind of touch he wants afterward, are one of the best ways you can show him your genuine affection.

The Glans Penis:
Head of the Snake

There are several highly receptive areas at the end of the tipili. The ridge that runs around the bottom of the head is called the corona. Just below this ring there is a little V-shaped spot called the frenulum. For many men this membrane, which is similar to the tissue underneath the tongue, is the most intensely pleasurable place on the whole tipili. For others, the glans or Head of the Snake itself is the most sensitive. For uncircumcised men, the foreskin and the areas of exposed skin underneath are highly sensitive. Another erogenous zone that is sometimes overlooked is around the opening where his pre-ejaculate comes out, at the tip of the tipili. Every man likes these areas stroked differently at different times during the various stages of his arousal.

Testicles:
Sacred Spheres of Life, Seed Carriers, or Sacred Jewels

The skin of the scrotum (testicles) is also sensitive to light touching and stroking. The Sacred Jewels of the scrotum may be quite ticklish. While some men enjoy generous attention with various kinds of kissing and stroking here, others may not. For some, especially after ejaculation, the testicles are too sensitive for even the lightest touch.

Perineum:
Sacred Valley of Pleasure

Males can also be aroused by light stroking and touching of the perineum (the area of soft tissue between the testicles and the anus). The prostate gland is another male erogenous zone that may be stimulated through firm pressure on the perineum or through the anus. Some men are not aware that the Sacred Valley of Pleasure is an erotic zone, and so, once again, it is important to find out the kind of pressure he likes here. Try gently stroking his Sacred Valley when he is near reaching climax, and see how he responds.

Anal Cavity:
Rear Cavern

See description on the Anal Cavity below for both women and men.

FEMALE EROGENOUS ZONES
OF PLEASURE

Watching the interplay between the erogenous zones of a woman is an amazing experience to behold. While she is becoming aroused, the Sacred Moth and Sacred Butterfly flutter, the Flying Serpent lifts its head in the Forest until it becomes engorged with blood. The Entrance

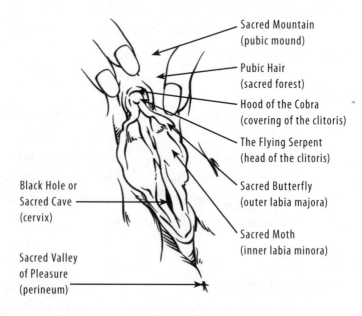

Fig. 6.2. The Tupuli, or Flying Feather Winged Serpent, otherwise known as the female sexual-creative organ, or the vulva (vagina)

beckons as her Sacred Cave pulses and thickens in wait. It is up to you to notice and play with the signals of delight her body shows you and to make her body sing with pleasure. Is there anything more beautiful than this? If you patiently watch for her responses, while you will never find a formula, her body will tell you things that she is hoping you will discover. It can be as simple as watching her neck arch, seeing the sway of her breasts, or noticing her thighs slightly part as a subtle clue to kiss her there.

The key to being a great lover is to pay attention to how your partner responds to the interplay between each of her pleasure zones. While it is true that women have different desires during their cycles, and usually dislike the same approach over and over again, there are several important places you should get to know well. While anywhere on a woman's body can be highly sensitive to touch, these are the erogenous zones to focus on. And as you will see in the next chapter, the position of these pleasure zones is different for each of the nine female genital anatomy types.

The Vagina:
The Sacred Tupuli

It could be said that the entire vulva is an erogenous zone, because sensuous touch anywhere inside, surrounding, and near the tupuli, when applied with great finesse, proper timing, and attention to what she likes, gradually arouses a woman into lovely states of delight. Always keeping in mind that even when you know the features of a woman's sexual anatomy and are familiar with her vagina, it is wise to continually watch for the movements of her body, listen to the sounds she makes, and to ask her what she prefers.

Entrance to the Sacred Cave

The Entrance to the Cave is not a specific anatomical part; it refers to the nerve-dense, elastic area at the entrance of the vagina. Right inside the vaginal opening, there is an internal band of sensitive muscular tissue. This ring of muscles, extending about an inch inside the vaginal tunnel, is particularly responsive for many women and deserves considerable attention.

The Flying Serpent: Head of the Clitoris

Most people think the clitoris is the knob of the vagina you can see perched between a woman's lips. The clitoris, or Flying Serpent, however, actually spreads out internally, branching out in two wings that extend into the vagina up along the pubic mound (Sacred Mountain). Because the internal "wings" are also dense with sensitive nerves, this entire area is highly sensitive when aroused. These two wings form a shaft, coming together to form the "head" or glans of the clitoris. The tip of the clitoris is a sensitive yet intensely pleasurable erotic zone for most women. Quodoushka calls it the Head of the Cobra.[1]

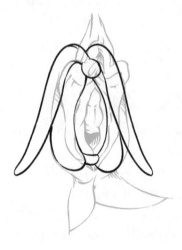

Fig. 6.3. The Flying Serpent (Entire Clitoris Region)

Some women's Flying Serpents are covered by a thick hood of skin that functions in a similar way to the foreskin of a penis. Others are lightly hooded or entirely exposed. The size of the Flying Serpent and position of the hooding also vary with each feminine anatomy type (see chapter 8), and thus different women prefer different types of stimulation. Generally, because a woman with very thin hooding has a more exposed clitoris, she is more sensitive and thus prefers light pressure, whereas a woman with a thicker covering usually likes stronger stimulation.

The G-Spot:
Secret Fire Trigger

The G-spot is not a modern invention. Ancient Chinese Taoists referred to this wonderful center of pleasure as Lute Strings, and Quodoushka calls it The Secret Fire Trigger of the Serpent, or, more simply, the Secret Fire Trigger. Both these names reflect something the term *G-spot* does not quite accurately convey: this area inside the vaginal tunnel, which is located at varying depths along the upper wall within the urethral sponge, is not a specific spot. It is a network of interconnected blood vessels and nerves. The tissue of this area is similar to the tissue of the prostate gland and to the frenulum underneath the rim of a man's tipili. When a woman is turned on, this area becomes engorged with blood, and the Secret Fire Trigger expands.

Scientists are still debating whether what has commonly become known as the G-spot exists as a distinct organ. Various sexual experts claim there is a female prostate gland located near the entrance of the vagina that is responsible for the copious amount of fluid women may produce during various forms of stimulation. Regardless of what this exciting research concludes in years to come, there is undeniably a highly pleasurable area located along the upper wall of the vaginal tunnel. While sexual experts and scientists may disagree on the purpose of female ejaculation, as women become more familiar with their Fire Triggers, they can have stronger orgasms, a significant increase of sexual secretions, and a great deal of pleasure exploring this erogenous zone.[2]

HOW TO FIND THE FIRE TRIGGER (G-SPOT)

As a lover, rather than searching for a stationary spot that can be turned on or off like a light switch, it is wise to approach the Secret Fire Trigger as an expanding and contracting zone of pleasure. Every woman has an area along the upper wall of her vagina that is highly sensitive, although some women are more aware of it than others. Before applying direct pressure here, however, it's best to enjoy some extended foreplay, gradually awakening her sensations by touching her face, her belly, her breasts, her neck, and her thighs before venturing to the inner and outer lips of her tupuli. If the Fire Trigger is prematurely touched, or too much pressure is applied before the blood has engorged the region, many women will experience discomfort rather than pleasure. Keep in mind that it is a woman's arousal that causes the nexus of nerve endings to converge into a place where you will find her Secret Fire Trigger.

When she is ready, if you take a finger or two and gently stroke the upper wall of her tupuli in a "come hither" motion, you will notice there is a place that has a different texture. Make sure you are both in comfortable positions so you can stay here and explore. As she continues to feel aroused, you should feel an area that is slightly more ridged than the surrounding tissue. Some describe it as being like a cat's tongue, although it is not as rough. You do not need to find an exact spot, so if you are not sure, don't worry. Once she begins to relax into the sensations, you can increase the pressure and speed on her Fire Trigger. Some

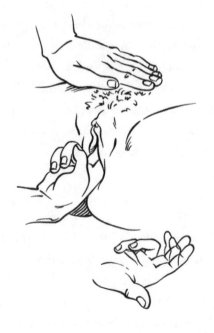

Fig. 6.4. Finding the Secret Fire Trigger (G-Spot Area)[3]

women like a lot of pressure here, or very fast motions, so find out what works best for her. Some women feel they have to urinate when being pleasured this way, but if you continue to explore the sensations, this feeling will subside.[4]

Depending on her sexual anatomy type, the Fire Trigger can be located quite close to the opening of her vaginal entrance, midway back, or it may be back further than a finger can reach. In a Deer Woman (explained in more detail in the next chapter), the Fire Trigger is located about a quarter of an inch inside the opening; whereas in a Dancing Woman, you may not be able to reach this erotic zone even by extending your fingers all the way inside her cave. For most of the other anatomy types, the Fire Trigger is located midway along the upper wall of her tupuli.

The Cervix:
The Sacred Black Hole

The cervix is located at the tip of the uterus at the very rear of a woman's tupuli. Excellent books now give guidance on how to see the cervix with a mirror, if you are so inclined.

During penetration some women enjoy repeated touch, whether by a finger or a tipili, along or under the rim of the Sacred Black Hole. For many, stroking around and entering the cervix during intense arousal is extremely pleasurable. Prolonged and loving touch in this zone can induce exceptionally ecstatic states of pleasure. However, you need to be careful by making sure there is plenty of lubrication, because this area can easily be bruised. Some women say that stimulation around the cervix can range from being mildly uncomfortable to painful. Changing positions, using more lubrication, being gentler, and making sure she is sufficiently turned on are good ways to discover the beauty of the Black Hole.

For these and any sexual explorations, it is extremely important to be exceptionally clean. Because bacteria can easily multiply in any of these erogenous zones for both men and women, it cannot be said enough how important using condoms when appropriate and practicing safe sex are for your health.

Quodoushka views each of these erogenous zones, including the Entrance to the Sacred Cave (opening), the Flying Serpent (clitoris), the Secret Fire Trigger (G-spot area), and the Black Hole (cervix), as equally erogenous and creates no hierarchy of orgasms. In other words, having a cervical orgasm (where the entire internal walls of the vaginal tunnel are stimulated and feel "full") is as intensely pleasurable as an orgasm primarily focused in the clitoral area. (See chapter 10, "The Nine Types of Orgasmic Expression.")

Perineum:
Sacred Valley of Pleasure

Located between the vaginal opening and the anal opening lies a fleshy patch of soft tissue. Lightly stroking this area in circular motions increases a woman's arousal toward climax. Most women will not climax as a result of perineum stimulation alone, but when combined with clitoral stimulation, orgasm is more readily achieved. While this region is stimulating for women, it especially pleasurable for men. When a woman presses her finger in the middle of the Sacred Valley of Pleasure right before and during her partner's release, it can lead to multiple climaxes.

The Anal Cavity:
The Rear Cavern

Although technically the anus is not part of the structure of the vagina (or penis) it certainly must be included as one of the erogenous zones. Much of this guidance applies to men as well. Many people say that anal sex increases the intensity of their orgasms. As with other erotic play, too much extreme focus on anal sex is not recommended. It is viewed more as an occasional, highly pleasurable erotic zone that can greatly intensify orgasms when you are in the mood.

To enter the Rear Cavern successfully, one must follow certain rules; the first is to never be too rough. Tearing the tissues inside or around the anus can lead to serious health problems and opens the door to infections and disease. Cleanliness is paramount. Never enter the anus and then touch inside or near the vagina. The simple rule is: wash thoroughly, even if it means interrupting sensuous play. The risks are too great for any exceptions.

Another important guideline that will make exploring the Rear Cavern pleasurable is to focus on the insertion. In other words, focus on the inward thrusts and then pull back gently. Do not pull out entirely from the Rear Cavern and then thrust inwards in rapid in and out motions. Focusing on the inward thrusts and more gentle withdrawals will eliminate any rips or tears inside the walls of the anal tunnel.

Taking great care to cleanse the area with warm water and a mild soap both before and afterward, using the proper type of thrusts, and making sure there is plenty of lubrication can make anal sex an extremely pleasurable experience for both men and women. While some may be able to reach orgasm through stimulation of the Rear Cavern alone, most people enjoy simultaneous stimulation of the tupuli or tipili. Arousing the genitals at the same time with your hands can produce particularly intense orgasms.

7

·OUR GENITAL ANATOMY

It is said that for us to know another, we must first know ourselves. When it comes to our most intimate, private parts, however, many of us spend a lifetime with only a vague appreciation of our own sexual anatomy. While we may have enjoyed many wonderful orgasms, we understand little about the way various vaginas and penises differ from one another and assume they are more or less the same. Once you learn about these genital anatomy types, you will never look at a penis or vagina in quite the same way again. While you can certainly get by knowing only the bare essentials about your genitals, when you know your anatomy type, a whole new world of sexual delight opens at your fingertips.

Hundreds of years ago, the Twisted Hairs Elders discovered that men and women could be categorized into nine different sexual anatomy types that describe in detail the effect your genital anatomy has on your sexual pleasure. Things such as how long it takes you to reach orgasm, how wet you become, how much you ejaculate, what you taste like, and whether you tend to like oral sex more than intercourse are greatly influenced by the position of the various erotic centers within and surrounding your genitals. For both men and women, your genital anatomy gives you insights into the reasons why you enjoy certain kinds of stimulation more than others. Remarkably, even things such as how you best attract part-

118

ners and initiate sexual encounters are all shaped by what kind of sexual anatomy you have.

From over twenty-five years of observing thousands of genitals, Quodoushka instructors have been able to observe the differences within each of the nine male and female genital anatomy types. Doctors and gynecologists who attend Quodoushka trainings have been fascinated by the following descriptions of genitalia and say there are no such classifications in the Western medical model. There are, however, other ancient sexual systems, including Hindu and Taoist anatomy teachings, that speak of various genital types. While they have different names than Quodoushka, these classifications were created to help people become skilled in the art of sensuous love.

THE GENITAL SENSE OF SELF

To better understand the significance of how our sexual anatomy type plays a role in our sexual expressions, it is important to realize we perceive everything around us through our gender. Quodoushka calls our fundamental gender orientation to life the Genital Sense of Self. "Is it a boy or a girl?" is the first thing parents ask. It is widely known that as bodies develop in the womb, both male and female fetuses touch their genitals for extended periods, which suggests that the sensations originating in their genitals are stronger than any others.

According to the shamanic view, a human spirit chooses its parents and its gender before birth. At the moment of conception, during the act of lovemaking, a great energy is released. It is the illumination and energy from this sexual act that attracts the spirit of the child to come into physical existence through a particular womb. Even with in vitro inseminations, the egg and semen are charged with orgasmic energy. Spirit has weight and thus when the spirit of the child enters the womb somewhere in the second trimester, the mother experiences a corresponding weight gain.

Well before we identify ourselves culturally, or within the context of a family, we choose our gender and perceive everything around us through our gender orientation. The countless messages we collect regarding our sexuality—both positive and negative—are absorbed into our bodies. Thus, when children are slapped for pleasuring their genitals, or are conditioned to feel ashamed about their own sexual sensations, it sets up tremendous confusion in the core of their Genital Sense of Self. Although our society is currently stretching the boundaries of what gender means, and some individuals are able to live more happily as they physically and emotionally change the appearance of their genders, how we feel about our genitals determines the way we experience pleasure and gain knowledge throughout our entire lives.

HEALING WOMEN'S GENITAL SHAME

This need for restoring a natural connection to the core of our sexuality is one of the reasons why the sexual anatomy wheels of Quodoushka are perhaps the most healing of all its teachings. When either men or women carry private doubts, fears, and insecurities about their genitals, it limits the energy they have available for everything else in life. Despite the abundance of sexual information available through books and websites, where pictures and labels describe various parts and techniques, understanding how to heal wounds in the Genital Sense of Self—or the way we *feel* about our own genitals—is largely absent.

Women seldom take the opportunity to carefully observe or get to know their own vulvas, and therefore many do not have a strong connection to their own sexual feelings. Few have any occasion or inclination to talk with other women about this subject, and most have never seen a variety of different vaginas. All this creates a perfect environment for shame to fester inside a woman's Genital Sense of Self. Even women who love sex may still fall prey to self-criticism or shame about the appearance of their vaginas. Some are convinced their lips are too large, too fleshy, or not the right color. Others worry whether too much self-pleasuring or childbirth has somehow changed the size or shape of their vaginas. While childbirth and aging do change the shape and appearance of the vagina over time, our sexual anatomy type remains the same. Self-pleasuring does not alter the shape of the lips.

When women are ashamed about their vaginas, it greatly limits their ability to enjoy sex. Not only can a woman's dislike of her own tupuli lessen her desire, the unfounded judgments, fears, and negative feelings that collect in her Genital Sense of Self *can* ultimately lead to cysts, unhealthy growths, and other illnesses. The main reason to know our sexual anatomy well is to heal our sexual sense of self and restore feelings of beauty and pride about our bodies. The following teachings about feminine anatomy serve to dispel prejudices regarding how women's vaginas are "supposed" to look. For many, it is a revelation to know there are such differences in feminine anatomy. Once a woman recognizes the uniqueness of her own genital anatomy, she can let go of unnecessary misconceptions and begin to appreciate the special magic of her sacred tupuli.

Most media images of genitals skew people's perceptions of themselves in subtly negative ways. The most common portrayals of genitalia in sexual magazines and movies depict small, petite vaginas for females, and large penises for males. The reality is, few of us actually look like what we see in the movies. In the same way we determine beauty based on what the media calls attractive, women frequently criticize their own genitals without ever realizing they have a certain type of sexual anatomy.

Yet when a woman learns she is a Buffalo Woman, for example, (whose lips protrude externally in fleshy, undulating folds), something begins to happen. Years of questions, doubts, and accumulated shame fall away. Relief, self-acceptance, and self-esteem soon follow, especially once she hears about the wonderful qualities a Buffalo Woman possesses. One gynecologist who recently attended Quodoushka shared the different types of tupulis with some of her clients who were considering cosmetic surgery because they did not like the way their vaginas looked. After she heard these teachings and saw the beauty of each different vagina type, she had an entirely different way of talking with clients who wanted to change the appearance of their tupulis.

With the permission of their parents, I have also introduced these sexual anatomy teachings to many young women. They were thrilled by the notion of being a Wolf or Cat, Dancing or Fox Woman, and they all wanted to know what type they were. When they found out, you could see how special they felt. They immediately took the animals to heart and started to dart around like cats and deer. But through their laughter and play, you could see a sense of secret joy set in, which more than likely later found its way into their love lives. It was something precious and dear for mothers and daughters to know about each other.

Sharing teachings about sexual anatomy is an incredibly empowering experience for women to learn about the unique qualities of their vaginas. When young women are introduced to these teachings properly, they gain respect for their own bodies and their own sexuality, and it gives them the confidence to choose what is right for them.

HEALING MEN'S GENITAL INSECURITY

Learning about the nine different genital anatomy types is profoundly healing for men too. Because their genitals are exposed, men typically look and touch them far more frequently than women touch theirs. Yet most men have mixed feelings about their penises. They alternate between feeling proud and vaguely inadequate. Comparing themselves to other men, they often think they are too small, or, in some cases, may even think they are too big.

Even though men can see other male genitalia in bathrooms or locker rooms, they don't want to seem overly interested, and so they become good at taking quick, furtive glances. Furthermore, they rarely see other men aroused and thus forget about the great difference in size between an erect and flaccid penis. The comparisons men make with their own genitals are not only inaccurate; their self-criticism undermines their sexual prowess. Women who think that men are relatively "fine" with their penises would be amazed at how shy and inadequate they often feel about their genitals. Many men consider the size of their penis as being the central factor in fully satisfying a woman, while in reality the size of a penis plays only a partial role in sexual pleasure. Turning around feelings of being flawed or somehow lacking is critical to assuring a man's sense of potency at the core of his sexual self.

A Note from a Bear Man

When I heard I was a Bear Man, I loved it. I think it "psychically" made me feel thicker, like I could somehow fill my partner better. I used to have fantasies like most men about having a huge cock like a Horse Man, and when I showered in the gym with the guys, I think I was one of the smallest. But now I realize that length is not as important as thickness. I think a lot of guys worry more about what other guys think and have big egos about their size, but that's not where it really counts. When the moment of truth comes, being a Bear Man works for me. In fact, now that I look back, I think a lot of girls were attracted to me because I was just being myself. Since then I have read different things about sexuality, and I know that certain positions are better for me. I learned how to move in different directions and use different strokes inside my lover. I know I can totally satisfy her as long as I give her everything I've got. That includes being more aware of what she likes instead of just thinking about myself. For me, it's all about learning to use what you have.

JIM

When a man understands his anatomy, he can learn how to take advantage of his best traits. Feeling self-assured about his penis affects just about everything he does. When a man accepts himself for who he is and discovers there are several things beyond size that can make him a good lover, he can develop his sexual skills in much more fulfilling ways. Most importantly, he must go beyond his own gratification and use his natural abilities to improve the quality of his love skills.

Quodoushka teaches that every anatomy type has distinct advantages. After viewing so many male and female genitalia over the years, I have come to see that while there are different categories, each one is unique. Furthermore, it is important to keep in mind that our anatomy is merely the starting point of our erotic potential. Once you learn the specific preferences and tendencies of your genital type, you are by no means limited to experiencing the attributes of one direction. In fact, with practice, anyone can cultivate sexual abilities from any place on the wheel to liberate their erotic nature.

DOES MY PARTNER HAVE
THE "RIGHT" ANATOMY?

Before we begin to describe the various physical attributes and emotional characteristics of each type, you should know that there are no perfect matches. Deer or Horse Men, for example, are not limited to being with any particular type of woman, and while there may be certain preferences, any type of man can learn how to be with any type of woman.

Female Genital Anatomy
The Sacred Tupuli: How Anatomy
Affects a Woman's Sexual Pleasure

Much of the way a woman experiences pleasure has to do with her anatomy. This is because the way a woman's erotic centers of arousal are positioned in relationship to each other determines how she prefers to be stimulated. The key to increasing a woman's enjoyment of sex has to do with knowing more about the external and internal features of her tupuli. Learning the nuances of woman's genital anatomy gives you valuable guidance on how to regularly bring her to the highest states of pleasure possible. You will discover how you can "play" each part of her sexual anatomy to make them sing together. At first, while you are getting to know the details, they may seem like separate places, but with practice you will see how the lips, the clitoris, the opening, and the Fire Trigger (G-spot area) are all connected.

Taking the time to find out about your partner's anatomy type gives you a way to explore the kinds of pressure, speed, and timing she likes best. You will also gain a better sense of when to change your touch and timing if something doesn't work for her. Remember, however, that there are no fixed formulas, and that you must always pay close attention to what she wants in any given moment. The best way to increase your sensitivity and skill as a lover is to be curious, ask questions, get feedback, and stay open for change.

A woman's genital anatomy type will tell you the approximate location of her Fire Trigger—whether it's close to the opening or much further back. It will tell you something about the depth of her cave, and thus will explain why she likes certain positions more than others. It will also give you insights about the time it takes her to reach orgasm, as well as the ways she likes to be approached for sexual play. Because many women do not know their own sexual anatomy well, it can be difficult for them to express what they need. Unfortunately, some women think there is something wrong because they are not feeling much pleasure with penetration. They may wonder why they are not well lubricated, or are worried that they take too long to climax. Understanding each other's anatomy answers these and many other questions about the styles of seduction that are most natural for us.

While we may know we are all sexually different from each other, what we don't know is how our anatomical features influence what we like and dislike. As you will see from the descriptions, the physical characteristics of a Deer Woman's genital anatomy, for example, cause her to prefer certain types of arousal more than others. Furthermore, her sexual demeanor is quite different than a Sheep Woman's and all the other types. The Deer Woman is quick and magically seductive, whereas a Sheep Woman has a sweet, emotional nature. It's an exciting adventure to find out what type of man or woman you are, and it will bring enduring insights into your love life for years to come.

8

FEMALE GENITAL ANATOMY TYPES

IDENTIFYING A WOMAN'S GENITAL ANATOMY

Have fun reading through the various descriptions of each type to see which one you think you are. To find your anatomy type, you might want to start by looking at the physical features of your tupuli by yourself using a mirror. It's also fun to consider the following descriptions and illustrations while looking in the mirror with a lover.

Because several of the physical characteristics used to determine a woman's genital type cannot be easily seen, whether you are looking by yourself or with a lover, you will need to consider both the internal and external features of the tupuli.

A Woman's Physical Genital Features

To identify a woman's sexual anatomy, first look at these external parts:

- the size and contour of the inner and outer lips
- the distance between the clitoris and the vaginal opening
- the shape of the hood covering the clitoris
- the overall size and shape of the entire vulva

Internally, try to determine:

- the depth and width of the vaginal cave (the average depth is about three-and-a-half inches in a relaxed state; some are somewhat shorter or longer, and they all expand when aroused)
- the location of the Fire Trigger/G-spot area (see chapter 6, "Locating the Fire Trigger," and fig. 6.4)

Other qualities that differ in feminine anatomy types include:

- the general taste of feminine secretions (all secretions vary with health and during a woman's cycles; the tastes listed with each type refer to a woman's healthy sexual secretions)
- the average time it takes to reach orgasm
- the typical amount of lubrication

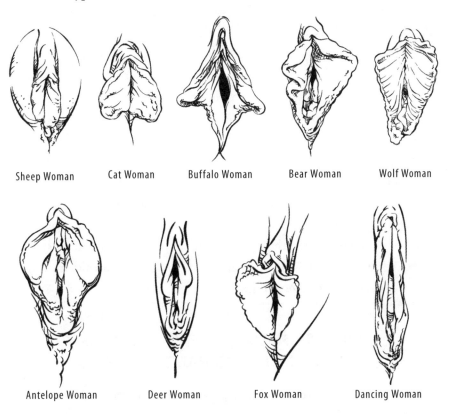

Sheep Woman   Cat Woman   Buffalo Woman   Bear Woman   Wolf Woman

Antelope Woman   Deer Woman   Fox Woman   Dancing Woman

Fig. 8.1. Nine Female Anatomy Types

How to Identify Your Type

If you would like to explore which type you are on your own, observe, explore, and enjoy learning more about yourself as you read through the sexual temperaments that go with each different anatomical type. One of the things that will help you determine your genital anatomy type is to look at the distance between the clitoris and the vaginal opening. (The distance is measured by a woman's own fingers, placed side by side, underneath the head of the clitoris. Thus, a Deer Woman's distance would only be the width of one finger, whereas a Dancing Woman's might be the width of four fingers.) Then try to find out where the Fire Trigger G-spot area is. Generally, if the head of the clitoris, the vaginal opening, and the Fire Trigger are located close together, then penetration will stimulate these three erogenous zones simultaneously. If the Fire Trigger, vaginal opening, and clitoris are further apart, then penetration alone will not stimulate these pleasure zones simultaneously. Thus, as you will see in the descriptions for each type, other kinds of sensuous play can be added to greatly increase a woman's pleasure.

As you identify which type you are, you may notice you have all the physical features of a certain direction, yet you do not have all the other qualities. Let's say you seem to be a Wolf Woman based on the physical descriptions, yet you do not like to make sounds as described. This means that you have the proclivity and the natural ability to easily let your voice go while making love. As you become more open and accepting of your sexuality, the inherent natural traits of your genital anatomy type will come forth. While even a Wolf Woman (or any of the anatomy types) may prefer at times to quietly express their lovemaking sounds, when you identify your anatomy type, you can use the descriptions to discover things about yourself that you may wish to bring out in yourself as a lover.

VARIETIES OF FEMALE GENITAL ANATOMY
AND THE NONCARDINAL DIRECTIONS

Each of the noncardinal directions (Southeast, Southwest, Northwest, and Northeast) has a combination of internal and external anatomical aspects of the two adjacent directions. For example, an Antelope Woman

(Northeast) will have some qualities of a Wolf Woman (North) and some of a Deer Woman (East). The types in the noncardinal directions also have some of the sexual demeanors and temperaments of the surrounding directions. This means a Northwest Bear Woman's orgasms will be heightened by both physical connections (West) and/or through fantasy and mental stimulation (North). Yet the noncardinal types are not only combinations of the attributes from either side. They also have the unique characteristics of the animal in that direction. Thus a (Southeast) Cat Woman has certain features of the South (Sheep) and East (Deer) directions, plus the unique demeanor associated with cats.

For both male and female types, you cannot be a combination of two types across the wheel. Thus, you cannot be a Wolf/Sheep Woman, or a Deer/Buffalo. Likewise, a man cannot be a Horse/Coyote or a Deer/Bear Man. Only the four cardinal directions (North, South, East, and West) and the two surrounding directions are used to determine the noncardinal types. The only exception is the Center direction. You can be

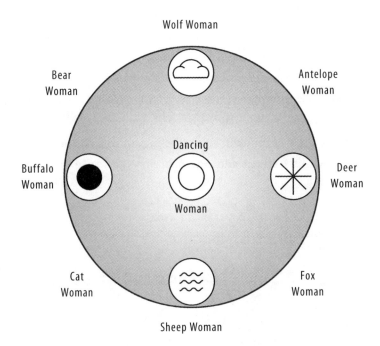

Fig. 8.2. Varieties of Female Genital Anatomy Types

a Dancing Sheep Woman (Center/South) or a Dancing Wolf Woman (Center/North) and so forth. A man can also be a Dancing Horse Man or Dancing Coyote Man, and so on.

SOUTH

Sheep Women

Sheep Women as Lovers

Modern sheep have evolved through thousands of generations of human contact. They are social creatures that stay close together for protection while grazing. Likewise, Sheep Women are gregarious, heart-centered women who find their strength by bonding in close-knit social clusters. Their demeanor is usually sweet and good-natured, yet they can become powerfully determined when something disturbs, frightens, or threatens them.

Sheep get agitated if they are not within eyesight of the flock. They have an innate instinct to go along with the group. Even if it's not a good idea, entire flocks will sometimes follow the leader over a cliff. However, they will also immediately warn fellow sheep of danger, and are extremely aware of the entire flock.

As lovers, Sheep Women have soft, compliant, and caring natures, yet they will also protect those they love without hesitation. These women have a natural ability to tune in to the feelings of others, and because their approach is usually indirect and gracious, they have an unusually disarm-

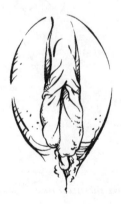

Fig. 8.3. Sheep Woman

ing way of affecting men with their sweetness. Their "soft power" can melt through overly aggressive or hasty advances. They tend to elicit their partner's gentler emotions during sex, but watch out, for when a Sheep Woman's heart is stirred, she awakens like a pounding thunderstorm.

Because they have a tendency to follow, Sheep Women need to learn to feel more comfortable leading and making independent decisions about what they desire. Their powerful emotions can overwhelm and confuse them, and they can easily lose sight of the importance of their own sexual needs and desires. When Sheep Women balance their emotional sensitivity and give pleasure to themselves as much as they give to others, they become exceptionally nurturing lovers.

Sheep Women are so naturally tuned in to emotions, they constantly challenge their lovers to express their feelings. They frequently desire deeper, more intimate heart connections, especially during sex. A Sheep Woman's orgasm is heightened to intense climax when her partner gives her tender caresses and loving words of endearment at just the right moments. If her partner arouses her in this way, and makes sure she feels completely safe and trusting, the force of her sex is like Niagara Falls. The sounds she makes during orgasms are called the Cries of Her Heart.

Distinguishing Features of Sheep Women

One of the distinguishing features of a Sheep Woman's genital anatomy is the long, tunnel-like hood that covers her clitoris. Another is the puffy, sometimes rounded shape of her vulva, which frequently has a distinctively rosy color. Sheep Women usually like rather vigorous stroking or sucking of the hooded tunnel that covers the clitoris, and thus they greatly enjoy oral sex. Sheep Women have particularly sweet-tasting secretions, and because they have a rather deep inner cave, they are also fond of extended, heartfelt intercourse.

Over the years, in speaking with many Sheep Women, we have found that they have a tendency to cry very easily, sometimes at the drop of a pin. As they sit in the South of the wheel, they respond emotionally, often with joyous laughter or even tears while making love. In addition, because the South is associated with water, they are almost always wet with sexual secretions—even if they are not aroused. Some Sheep Women describe being embarrassed by this. However, when Sheep Women accept their natural fluidity, they come to cherish the sweet wetness of their unique tupulis.

Summary of Sheep Women

Direction on the Wheel: South, the place of emotions, water, and giving with tenderness

Distance Between Clitoris and Vaginal Opening: Two to three fingers (place your fingers together horizontally right underneath the clitoris; for the Sheep Woman, there will be room for two to three fingers between the clitoris and the entrance to her cave)

Shape or Size of Hood: Long, smooth tunnel that entirely covers the clitoris

Inner Lips (Moth): Fairly thin lips (thicker and larger than a Deer Woman's)

Size of Cave: Fairly deep, five to seven inches

Location of Fire Trigger (G-spot Area): Fairly deep, midway back or deeper

Lubrication: Very wet

Temperature: Very cool

Taste: Sweet

Typical Time to Reach Orgasm: Fifteen to twenty minutes on average

Types of Stimulation: Enjoys lots of foreplay and oral sex, hard sucking, squeezing on the sides of the shaft of the clitoris and sliding back and forth, likes pubic mound grinding, very emotional, needs a heart connection to experience the fullness of her orgasms.

Types of Orgasm: Implosive, explosive waves. An implosive orgasm produces an orgasmic wave that moves inward, often causing the body to curl up in a fetus-like position. An explosive orgasm produces an orgasmic wave that moves outward, often causing the back, head, and arms to arch and reach outward.

Preferred Intercourse Positions: Woman on top, doggie style with bowed back, side to side with partner's legs between her legs

Preferred Male Anatomy Types: Likes Coyote Men because she enjoys grinding (enjoys other types as well)

Sexual Demeanor: Gregarious, inviting, heart-centered, sensitive, and deeply caring

SOUTHWEST

Cat Women

Cat Women as Lovers

Cats are some of the best hunters on the planet. It is a mistake, however, to see the generations of their domestication, often living in harmony with humans for many years, as being a sign of their total docility. If you observe a house cat chase and then pounce on a bird or watch it capture a mouse, you will clearly see its instinctual skills as a fierce hunter have not been lost.[1]

As lovers, Cat Women are no less fascinating and marvelous to behold. Although they are great fighters, they are also undeniably beautiful, affectionate, and soft. Like some cats that are so lithe and supple

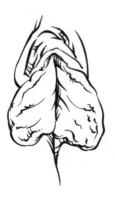

Fig. 8.4. Cat Woman

you can't take your eyes off them, Cat Women are true exhibitionists, although they often seem demure and shy at first. It's not that they like to brashly show off; rather, in certain moments of tender intimacy, when they feel totally safe and secure, they will allow their beauty to be seen with a kind of sophisticated, regal pride.

Once they make up their minds to go after something or someone they desire, Cat Women do not hesitate. When they apply this determined quality to their sexuality and learn to fully embrace their highly orgasmic natures, they are the most majestic, confident, and giving lovers of all the anatomy types. This self-assured, unselfish type of sexual giving (that they share with Sheep Women) makes their lovers swoon with gratitude and respect in their presence. A Cat Woman's purrs and roars are called her Secrets of Self-Love.

Like cats, these women can seem picky and aloof, bestowing their affections only when and on whom they prefer. In reality, cats are not actually aloof; they simply like to be alone at times, and like to rest in dark, quiet places. Cat Women are highly discerning and extremely sensitive about what they want in any given moment. They are particularly sensitive to the smell, taste, and touch of their partners. If you want to charm and arouse a Cat Woman, give her plenty of space. Let her know you adore and desire her, but then withdraw. Let the timing of when you get together be hers. Keep in mind that while she likes independence, she does not like to be ignored. Cat Women yearn for a secure place to express the wildness of their soft, receptive natures.

Just as cats do not attack their prey head-on but like to pounce from the rear, Cat Women can be sneaky. They frequently hold onto and lick their resentments for a long while and would rather avoid straightforward confrontations. They are often indirect and elusive to the point that they get confused about what they actually want. Cat Women easily get hooked on self-doubt, letting insecurities about their bodies interfere with their need for sexual expression. Their greatest challenge is to honestly, openly, and directly share their sexual needs and desires with their partners. When Cat Women learn to use their instinct of knowing when it's the right time to wait patiently and when it's time to take action, they transcend their fears and self-doubts to become passionately sensuous lovers.

Distinguishing Features of Cat Women

Like all the noncardinal anatomy types, Cat Women have characteristics of the adjacent types to the South and West. They have a mixture of Sheep (South) and Buffalo Women (West) characteristics. Cat Women have a pronounced hooding covering the entire clitoris, whose shaft is shorter than that of a Sheep Woman's. In addition, the upper part of a Cat Woman's outer lips is connected to the hood. (In all other types except for the Sheep, the hood covering the clitoris is a separate fold of skin that is not connected to the lips. In both Sheep and Cat Women, the hood and the lips are connected in one piece of skin.)

There is also a noticeable thickness or puffiness of the outer labia of a Cat Woman, yet they are less full and richly folded than a Buffalo Woman's lips. Her lips are often smaller in size than a Sheep Woman's. Sometimes Cat Women have what we call a double hood, meaning that they have two similarly sized folds of skin, one covering the clitoris, and then another hood hanging below. According to Quodoushka, this only occurs in Cat Women. Internally, Cat Women have shallower inner caves than Sheep Women, and they enjoy extended oral play as much as intercourse.

Summary of Cat Women

Direction on the Wheel: Southwest, the place of dreams, symbols, and adventure

Physical Features: A Cat Woman has physical and emotional characteristics of both Sheep Women (South) and Buffalo Women (West) (see surrounding descriptions of lips, size of hood, etc.); Cat Women may have internal features of the Sheep Woman, and external features similar to a Buffalo Woman, or vice versa; her sexual preferences are also a combination of the West and South directions

Sexual Temperament: Independent, gently affectionate, sweetly seductive, elusive, and unpredictable

WEST

Buffalo Women

Buffalo Women as Lovers

Buffalos, considered by Native Americans to be sacred, are the keepers of medicine and abundance because every part of their hides and meat has been used to feed and sustain the people for thousands of years. Lakota legends speak of a pure white buffalo that came to the tribe, turned into a woman, and taught humans how to live in harmony with nature. She became known as the beloved White Buffalo Calf Woman.

As lovers, Buffalo Women bring an easygoing, soothing presence into their relationships. They are straightforward in their approach to sex, and they revel in the earthly delights of lovemaking. They have powerful sex drives and are transported to the heavens through pure physical passion. These women like to be grazed upon for days. If you want to attract and court a Buffalo Woman, make sure you comment on the beauty of her body, and touch her often with affection. To open herself sexually, she desires and needs to feel your earthy body warmth and presence.

Then slowly, as things heat up and her sexual forces gather inside, watch out—because the stampede is coming. A Buffalo Woman likes to start leisurely, slowly, and delicately. Then, as her pleasure mounts, she will draw you to her until she finally expresses the full force of her orgiastic* joy with amazing power. During or right before orgasm, she will often wrap her legs around you tightly, pull you close, and then bite or fiercely kiss anywhere she can. Her orgasms are brought to a peak through physical sensations and connected touch. The sounds a Buffalo Woman makes during her orgasms are called the Songs of the Earth.

Courting a Buffalo Woman can be unpredictable and mysterious, for while she has a tendency to be forthright, honest, and direct about what

---

Orgiastic means "an excited, heightened state of awareness." While the word *orgiastic* is often used pejoratively to mean a state of wild, unconscious frenzy, or an orgy, Quodoushka uses the word in a positive manner, to indicate a state of heightened pleasure in the mind, which then excites the body. *Orgasmic* refers to the body's ability to physically experience orgasm; whereas *orgiastic* refers to the creative passion we experience during intense states of pleasure.

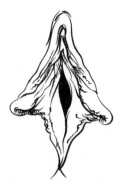

Fig. 8.5. Buffalo Woman

she wants, she can quickly change her mind. Typically, you will know when a Buffalo Woman wants to make love, because she will tell you. At times, however, her straightforward approach to lovemaking can be too much. As lovers, Buffalo Women must use their intuition to feel into the needs of others while learning to be more thoughtful, sensitive, and nuanced in their approaches to sex and intimacy. When Buffalo Women access their ability to tune into the human body, they instinctively feel their lovers' deep sexual needs. Like the buffalo, who gives away every part of itself to sustain life, Buffalo Women are intuitive, giving lovers who can use the extraordinary potency of their sexual love to heal themselves and others.

Distinguishing Features of Buffalo Women

One of the distinguishing features of a Buffalo Woman's genital anatomy is her large, protruding, thick outer lips, which curl and hang downward in cascading layers of skin. Some women may feel embarrassed about their large lips, but once they learn that many lovers enjoy sucking and tasting these sumptuous, earthy folds, they take great pride in being Buffalo Women.

Other distinct features of a Buffalo Woman's anatomy are the somewhat wide entrance and shallow depth of her vaginal cave. She must find positions that give her a good angle during intercourse so that she does not experience pain during deeper thrusts. One position that works well is with her legs held together so that she can control the depth of her lover's penetrations with her thighs. Once a Buffalo Woman is aroused and finds good positions, the depth and power of her inner cave expands.

Summary of Buffalo Women

Direction on the Wheel: West, the place of the body, Earth, holding and transforming with intimacy

Distance Between Clitoris and Vaginal Opening: Two to three fingers

Shape or Size of Hood: "Tepee-like," with many hanging folds

Inner Lips (Moth): Very thick, wrinkled, and protruding

Size of Cave: Shallow, three to five inches deep; wide, two to three inches in diameter

Location of Fire Trigger (G-spot area): Midway back (about two joints of a finger)

Lubrication: Moderately wet

Temperature: Very cool

Taste: Salty or earthy

Typical Time to Reach Orgasm: Fifteen to twenty minutes on average

Types of Stimulation: Enjoys a very slow pace until she nears climax; lots of foreplay, likes gentle rubbing of the folds on either side of the clitoris, strong sucking and licking of lips, sometimes underneath the hood, loves oral sex, pubic grinding, lots of sensuous play before, during, after orgasm

Types of Orgasm: Many earthquake-like, implosive orgasms; likes to hold, squeeze, kiss, or bite during orgasms

Preferred Intercourse Positions: Woman on top, doggie style with bowed back, side to side with partner's legs between her legs

Preferred Male Anatomy Types: Likes a Bear Man because his tipili is thick, but she enjoys others as well

Sexual Demeanor: Lusty, playful, direct, passionate, and powerfully sexual

NORTHWEST

Bear Women

Bear Women as Lovers

Female bears are physically powerful, yet for the most part they shy away from people and can be easily frightened. They guard their cubs in tucked-away places of warmth and safety. When a mother feels her cubs are in danger, she will ferociously defend them and will face any opponent who dares to threaten their lives. As lovers, Bear Women have vigilant, protective natures. They relish the fleshy, body feelings of sex like Buffalo Women, and they have quick minds like Wolf Women.

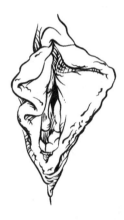

Fig. 8.6. Bear Woman

Lest you think bears only live in caves, however, never forget their fondness for climbing trees. Similar to a Buffalo Woman, a Bear Woman's sexual pace can be luxuriously slow, but then, as her excitement rises, she can climb quickly with unstoppable speed. It is wise to give all bears a wide berth, because they can be rather unpredictable. If you want to court a Bear Woman, get to know her typical patterns of arousal. Learn the sequence of what she finds stimulating by finding the timing of when she likes to go inward and when she is ready to take off for deeper pleasure. Once she has the physical closeness she needs, then surprise her with something she doesn't expect. Make sure you cuddle, hold her, and talk intimately after lovemaking.

Bear Women must carefully observe the timing of their hibernations, or they can become too reclusive and slide into the sleep of depression. They need to know when to withdraw and when to come out of their dens to play and make love. A Bear Woman's greatest challenge is to let go of overly protective defenses, mellow her tempestuous nature, and use her power to manifest her creative talents in the light of day.

During lovemaking, a Bear Woman pulls her partner deeply into semiconscious states of dreaming. Her postcoital love naps strengthen primal instincts and can invoke the magic and mystery of unending sexual desire. She has quite an intoxicating effect on men, and she often likes to make love again after a rest. The thrust of her orgasms sweeps away all distractions, taking her lovers into unknown dimensions of erotic joy. The music of her moans is called the Longing of the Magical Dream.

Distinguishing Features of Bear Women

The lips of a Bear Woman are thick like those of the Buffalo Woman and may take the shape of butterfly wings like the lips of a Wolf Woman. They are somewhat less plush than the labia of a Buffalo Woman. They have almost as great a distance from the clitoris to the vaginal opening as in Dancing Women, and their Fire Trigger is fairly far back. They thus tend to enjoy deep thrusts during intercourse once they are really aroused. Finding the right pace, timing, and depth is essential for pleasing a Bear Woman.

Although some Bear Women's vaginal caves are fairly deep as in a Wolf Woman, some are as shallow as a that of a Buffalo Woman. Like the Buffalo and Wolf, a Bear Woman likes different positions. During her rise to climax, she may wish to bring her legs together to guide the depth of penetrations. Then she may enjoy changing to doggie style during intercourse.

Summary of Bear Women

Direction on the Wheel: Northwest; the place of pattern, timing, and the Sacred Body Image

Physical Features: Bear Women have characteristics of both Wolf Women (North) and Buffalo Women (West); they may have internal features of the Wolf Woman and external features similar to a Buffalo Woman, or vice versa; their sexual preferences and temperament are also a combination of the West and North directions

Sexual Demeanor: Affectionate, protective, secretive, alternately shy and powerfully sexual[2]

NORTH

Wolf Women

Wolf Women as Lovers

As hunters, wolves cover vast areas, tracking prey using their acute senses of hearing, sight, and smell. While they hunt both by day and night, they are commonly thought of as wild nocturnal animals howling at the moon. As lovers, Wolf Women establish their territories by quickly tuning in to their attractions. Upon entering a room of people, they immediately scan to see who they find most intriguing.

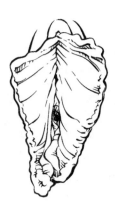

Fig. 8.7. Wolf Woman

Wolf Women sit in the North of the Medicine Wheel and are thus associated with the mind. Like wolves, who have complicated systems of facial and body gestures along with a variety of meaningful growls, barks, and yelps, Wolf Women are highly intelligent, reflective, and often witty communicators. Stimulating conversation turns them on, and it is an important part of their foreplay ritual. They love fantasies, sexy talk, and humor before, during, and after sex. If you want to court a Wolf Woman, make sure you stimulate her mind first. Wolf Women love to moan and howl during sex. Her wonderful screams of ecstasy are called Songs of the Moon.

Interestingly, some who find out they are Wolf Women tell us they don't make much noise during sex. This may be due to social conditioning that did not give them permission to voice ecstatic bliss. However, when a quieter Wolf Woman learns this is her natural inclination, she can release uninhibited cries of pleasure if she wants to. In my observation, the sounds a woman makes during lovemaking are very personal. Whether she roars loudly, or quietly moans, what matters most is that she feels free to do whatever she likes. For most women, but especially a Wolf Woman, the moans of delight vibrating through her body during sex intensify her passion and set free the full expression of her orgasmic joy.

In the Sweet Medicine Sundance teachings, the wolf is known as the "keeper of the path with heart." This is because wolves govern themselves in clear hierarchies within the pack and frequently mate for life. As lovers, Wolf Women are loyal, devoted partners. They like to hunt for stimulating friendships, yet at times value their independence like lone wolves. Wolf Women are alternately intense, feisty, and playful and are good at bringing unusual, spicy ideas into their bedrooms.

Because Wolf Women can become caught in their own minds, they tend to overthink things until their cleverness gets the best of them. They need to enter into the deeply calm, quiet spaces of sensual love more often where they can let go, trust their instincts, and be more spontaneous. When they move with the flow of their erotic feelings, get out of their heads and into their bodies, the power of their sexual intelligence flourishes with astonishing grace. Whenever she directs the quickness of her mind to pure passion, her orgasms can whip through all time, space, and dimensional realities.

Distinguishing Features of Wolf Women

The most noticeable physical feature of a Wolf Woman is the shape of her tupuli lips. If you pull apart her outer lips, they take the shape of smooth, thin butterfly wings. Sometimes one is larger than the other. Frequently, internally, Wolf Women have tipped uteruses and often say they feel as if they need to urinate (because they feel pressure against their bladder) during intercourse. Shifting positions can change this feeling of pressure. Also, it's best to make sure the bladder is empty before making love.

Another common trait Wolf Women report is their fondness for making love during or near their menstruation (when they are sometimes known to "howl at the moon" in pleasure). Her strong affinities to the cycles of the moon bring out her desire for intimacy, sex, and love.

Summary of Wolf Women

Direction on the Wheel: North, the place of the mind, wind, and receiving

Distance Between Clitoris and Vaginal Opening: One to two fingers on average

Shape or Size of Hood: Slight or average hooding covering the clitoris

Inner Lips: Fairly large, smooth, thin, butterfly-shaped

Size of Cave: Moderately shallow, four to five inches deep, 1⅛ to 1¼ inches in diameter

Location of Fire Trigger (G-spot Area): Somewhat back, variable; this area may give a sense of bladder pressure when it is stimulated

Lubrication: Wet

Temperature: Warm to hot

Taste: Sweet-salty

Typical Time to Reach Orgasm: Twenty to thirty minutes on average

Types of Stimulation: Enjoys strong oral and clitoral stimulation once she is aroused, likes slow or hard grinding, steady pace with "head popping" (entirely withdrawing the head of the penis from the vagina and then re-inserting the head during intercourse), then strong and fast during climax; heightened arousal during or near menstruation; windlike, intense orgasms; enjoys stimulating conversations and fantasy

Types of Orgasm: Explosive-implosive. As stated earlier, an implosive orgasm produces an orgasmic wave that moves inward, often causing the body to curl up in a fetus-like position. An explosive orgasm produces an orgasmic wave that moves outward, often causing the back and head to arch, or the arms to reach outward.

Preferred Intercourse Positions: Likes most except high leg positions

Preferred Male Anatomy Types: Likes many types, especially Dancing Men and Deer Men; sometimes Horse Men can be too large

Sexual Demeanor: Intelligent, insightful, wild, creative, and intense

NORTHEAST

Antelope Women

Antelope Women as Lovers

Antelopes have some of the mental agility of wolves and the magic of deer. They are one of the great migratory animals that love to run. In

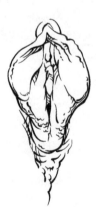

Fig. 8.8. Antelope Woman

the Medicine Wheel, they sit in the place of energy design and are thus known for being dance-like choreographers. As lovers, they are sensuous artists in motion who captivate partners with poised elegance and nimble grace. They are naturally flirtatious and nearly hypnotic in their ability to seduce. Antelope Women have an innate flair for adventure in their relentless pursuit of pleasure and knowledge. They are intensely passionate, focused, and uninhibited lovers who yearn to express their creative passions.

Unlike sheep or cats that thrive in captivity, antelope immediately try to escape if they are fenced in, sometimes hurting themselves in the process. Not a single species of antelope or gazelle has ever been domesticated. Similarly, an Antelope Woman has a disdain for being corralled into routine. She has a need to express her imagination, and she flourishes by having multiple sexual attractions. When her cries of bliss rise from deep within her body, they are called the Songs of Heaven.

In pursuit of a predator or during play, antelope do something called pronging, in which they jump into the air by lifting all four feet off the ground simultaneously. Antelope Women are thus known as "jumpers" because what takes them over the edge sexually is change. While making love to an Antelope Woman, you need to vary your speed, positions, and types of touch. If you change at just the right moments (she likes to be surprised) and quicken or slow your pace in the midst of sexual play, the "jumps" will take her to pleasure peaks where she can finally surrender.

If you want to charm and arouse an Antelope Woman, do the unexpected. (While this works for almost all women, it works especially well for Antelopes.) Take her into the silence of burning love, bring her something rare, bizarre, or funny, and show her things she does not know about herself. If you can find the secret passions hidden in her whirling vortexes, she will let go of her erotic juices for you.

An Antelope Woman's biggest challenge is to enjoy incremental, gradual changes. Rather than determining that lovers or situations are boring and predictable, they benefit by resisting the temptation to flee and by staying close to those they love. Antelope Women are prone to being divided and stuck between seemingly opposing desires. When they listen to their instincts before leaping into things, Antelope Women boldly initiate the changes they seek. In this way, Antelope Women have ingenious ways of enticing their partners into joyful moments with their free and easy power.

Distinguishing Features of Antelope Women

In their orgasmic patterns, Antelope Women have the quickness of Deer Women and thus have the capacity to reach multiple orgasms. (All women have this capacity, but Antelope and Deer Women can access it more easily.) They also have the intelligence, imagination, and intensity of Wolf Women. Physically, an Antelope woman's lips are somewhat thin and delicate like the Deer Woman's, but they spread to appear like small butterfly wings like the Wolf Woman's. Internally, the Antelope Woman can be fairly deep like the Deer; her Fire Trigger is about midway back, and she goes from being sometimes dry at arousal to extremely juicy. A unique physical characteristic of the Antelope Woman is the long distance (about four to five fingers) between her anal opening and her vaginal opening. Typically, she also has wrinkles surrounding her anus.

Summary of Antelope Women

Direction on the Wheel: Northeast; place of focus, relaxation, and design of energy

Physical Features: Has characteristics of both Wolf Women (North) and Deer Women (East); Antelope Women may have internal features of the Wolf Woman and external features similar to a Deer Woman, or vice versa

Sexual Demeanor: Gracefully uninhibited, fun, imaginative, creative "jumpers" with adventurous spirits

EAST

Deer Women

Deer Women as Lovers

There are many stories of deer luring kings and hunters deep into the woods until they were lost and had to use mystical charms to find their way home. Buddha is often depicted with a deer by his side and is said to have embodied their gentle nature.[3] In the Sweet Medicine teachings, the deer is the Keeper of Magic. Wild deer have exceptionally fine senses of smell, hearing, and sight. They mark their territory by leaving a strongly scented pheromone that they secrete at the front of each eye. As lovers, Deer Women's beauty, innocence, and grace make them exquisite companions. They magically enchant their lovers and are known for creating intoxicating spells with their marvelously soft and elegant natures. If there is one word that captures the unique allure of a Deer Woman, it would have to be *irresistible*.

Like deer running through the forests and nibbling on only certain leaves, Deer Women have delicately refined tastes. Because of their discerning preferences, they can be overly picky and critical. They are easily distracted and can shut down entirely if they sense something is not just right. Deer Women get turned on in a flash with

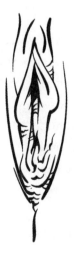

Fig. 8.9. Deer Woman

remarkable agility. They can often reach orgasm in less than a minute, and their buoyant alertness gives them magnetic powers and deft skills in the arts of love. Yet, if a Deer Woman wants to enjoy the subtler sensations of sex, she should learn to slow her movements and harness her quickness in order to extend her orgasmic pleasures. When she does slow down, she can finally bask in the full splendor of her amazing sensuous feelings.

Deer Women sit in the East of the Medicine Wheel, the place of fire and spirit. They desire spiritual communion in the rituals of passion, and they long to visit beautiful places for sacred ceremonies where they can linger in the glory of blissful union. If you want to successfully attract and arouse a Deer Woman, create an exalted atmosphere for love's complete expression, and then cherish her with absolute reverence.

In Chinese medicine, deer antlers are ground into powder for restorative remedies. They contain the fastest-growing tissues on Earth and are thus believed to confer sexual youth, endurance, and sexual potency. Deer Women can be long-term, fiercely loyal lovers who truly enjoy hot sex. They can lure their partners to surrender into the mystical realms of infinite rapture. Their moans of surrender and joy are called the Whispers of the Goddess.

Distinguishing Features of Deer Women

There are a number of distinguishing features of a Deer Woman's genital anatomy, which together combine to make her tupuli special and unique. The first are her extremely thin and tiny outer lips. In some cases, the entire length of her vulva can be less than an inch in length. These are the idealized vaginas most commonly depicted in pornographic magazines and movies. It is unfortunate so many women pick up the false idea that their own genitals are supposed to appear petite like the Deer Woman's, and sometimes undergo surgery to rectify the perceived discrepancy.

Nonetheless, the beautiful appearance of her tiny vulva is somewhat deceptive, as the Deer Woman has the deepest inner cave of all the anatomy types. Her Fire Trigger is located right inside the entrance of her vaginal opening and close to her clitoris. As a result, she can reach orgasm quickly, often with just a few strokes. She may easily have multiple orgasms and tends to prefer deep thrusts of extended intercourse. A Deer Woman typically becomes hotter and drier the more aroused she gets. Her barely covered, exposed clitoris is extremely sensitive. Thus, some say they do not enjoy strong oral sex or heavy grinding pressure on their pubic mounds. They can get sore if enough care is not taken during prolonged lovemaking and often like to use lubricants. As with all the other types, Deer Women can come to love oral sex and enjoy just about any lovemaking position.

Summary of Deer Women

Direction on the Wheel: East, the place of the fire, spirit, imagination, and determination

Distance Between Clitoris and Vaginal Opening: Clitoris and opening are right next to each other, less than a quarter-inch apart

Shape or Size of Hood: Barely hooded, sometimes exposed, tiny clitoris

Inner Lips (Moth): Very thin, small lips

Size of Cave/Entrance: Very deep, seven to nine inches, with tight entrance, three quarters of an inch to an inch diameter at opening

Location of Fire Trigger (G-spot Area): Right inside the Sacred Cave, easily reached; about a quarter of an inch up to a half an inch along the upper wall

Lubrication: Dry, although she can ejaculate (as can any anatomy type)

Temperature: Very hot

Taste: Sweet-tart

Typical Time to Reach Orgasm: One to three minutes on average

Types of Stimulation: Typically does not like much foreplay; direct oral and clitoral stimulation needs to be extremely gentle; because the clitoris is so sensitive and close to the cave's entrance, can become overstimulated or even irritated without sufficient lubrication; likes hard, fast, and deep thrusting and extended intercourse

Types of Orgasm: Fast, explosive; is aroused by spiritual, charismatic connections

Preferred Intercourse Positions: Likes them all, especially those with high leg positions

Preferred Male Anatomy Types: Likes many types, especially the Deer and Horse; has trouble with Coyote because of size

Sexual Demeanor: Enchanting, alluring, swift, hot, and magically seductive

SOUTHEAST

Fox Women

Fox Women as Lovers

Many shamanic legends from various traditions portray foxes as clever shape-shifters who can change into the form of seductive maidens. They are often depicted in folk tales as having cunning, mischievous, and supernatural powers, which they use to escape danger. Perhaps this is because foxes are seldom seen in the day and usually come out in what are

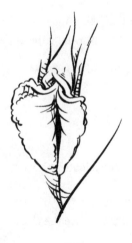

Fig. 8.10. Fox Woman

called the "cracks between the worlds." At twilight or dawn they can be seen darting back to their dens tucked away among rock crevices.[4] In our language, a "foxy lady" is a woman who has tantalizing ways of charming and seducing anyone she likes. The combination of her feminine wiles, of being resourceful and clever along with being dainty and graceful, make Fox Women unusually sexy. They are like love sirens tempting their lovers to enjoy the whole courtship, dance, and fun of sex.

A fox's style of solitary hunting describes the way Fox Women like to seduce their partners. Foxes hunt by patiently lying camouflaged, waiting for just the right moment to pounce. Likewise, Fox Women will often hold back at first, and then turn on their seductive charms at the perfect time. Calling a Fox Woman a tease would be an understatement (in a good way, of course). If you want to pique her curiosity, you must discover the subtle signs of her interest. She approaches sex indirectly, yet she will give you discrete little clues when she wants you to come closer. Like a magician whose magic is spoiled by too much direct exposure, a Fox Woman is at her best when mystery prevails. Her tempting, mesmerizing murmurs of love are called her Cries of Beauty.

In the Sweet Medicine Sundance path, the fox is the keeper of the family, because foxes are known to mate for life, and they return year after year to groom their cozy dens. Characteristically, like a gorgeous fox-tail, the demeanor of Fox Women is soft, hot, and cuddly. Despite their reputation for being the great seducers, they are actually sweet-natured, shy partners who are family-oriented, faithful lovers.

The greatest challenge for Fox Women is to stay focused and take their time. Like the fox that is attracted to shiny things and often loses its prey because it is enamored by the sight of its own tail, Fox Women are sometimes self-absorbed, perplexed, and easily distracted. Especially during lovemaking, when the slightest word, gesture, or even their own thoughts pull them away, they must learn to relax and enjoy what is happening. Self-love is the secret to being a truly foxy lady, for when a Fox Woman cherishes her own body, the sincerity and warmth of her affection will dazzle you with its radiant beauty. Her spontaneous generosity springs forth naturally whenever she feels truly loved.

Distinguishing Features of Fox Women

To recognize the physical features of a Fox Woman's genital anatomy, look at both the internal and external qualities of Sheep and Deer Women. The shaft of the Fox Woman's clitoral hooding is shorter than a Sheep Woman's. Her lips are petite, and her opening is close to her clitoris, yet her G-spot area is further back than a Deer Woman's. She can reach a climax in minutes or take much longer. She can become drier through arousal, or she can be profusely wet. Because a Fox Woman's sexual intimacy is enhanced by both a spiritual (East) and an emotional heart connection (South), she loves basking in the afterglow of sexual love.

Summary of Fox Women

Direction on the Wheel: Southeast is the place of self-love, self-concepts, attitude, and approach

Physical Features: A Fox Woman has characteristics of both Sheep Women (South) and Deer Women (East); Fox Women may have internal features of the Sheep Woman (fairly deep cave) and external features similar to a Deer Woman (small outer lips), or vice versa

Sexual Temperament: Friendly, loyal, unpredictable, and mischievously seductive

CENTER

Dancing Women

Dancing Women as Lovers

Dancing Women represent human beings in the full spectrum of their truth and beauty. Placed in the center of the Medicine Wheel, they alternately possess qualities of each direction. At times a Dancing Woman can be friendly and emotional like a Sheep Woman. Other times she revels in physical lust and likes to squeeze her lover tight like a Buffalo Woman. She possesses the mental quickness of the Wolf and the sexy charm of the Deer. Dancing Women love having options and open possibilities for sex. They can be chatty or quiet, teasing or compliant. They like to be challenged and will play hard to get, testing to see if you will pursue. They can be erotically spicy one minute and have you laughing the next.

Dancing Women are often the most secretly sexy of all the anatomy types, and though they might resist with shyness, when you find the key to their heart, they are warm, imaginative, and totally playful lovers. If you want to court a Dancing Woman, be especially persistent in letting her know how much you want her. Never take your eyes off her when you are making love to her. Try to bring out her kinky side from time to time. If you are relentless in your desire, she will reward you with her sweet surrender and give you a taste of sexual abandon. Dancing Women yearn to express their wisdom and long to feel their sexual power rippling throughout their bodies. When a Dancing Woman reaches orgasm, the sounds she makes are called her Cries of Freedom.

When she is in the mood, she can be as foxy as any Fox Woman and as slinky as a Cat Woman. Yet Dancing Women tend to dance around the wheel so much they can get lost in the maze of their own busyness. They are prone to doubt and have a hard time knowing what they want. The challenge for a Dancing Woman is to go for what she truly needs in

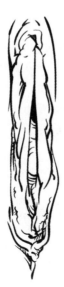

Fig. 8.11. Dancing Woman

any given moment. When she is honest about her vulnerability, allows her yearning for intimacy to be known, and values herself as a sexy, passionate woman, she is capable of changing anything. Because they have overcome great challenges in their romantic lives, Dancing Women are courageous spirits who have the capacity to play whatever roles their partners need. By their willingness to dive into the mysterious sides of sex, they inspire their lovers to freely express the beauty of their deepest desires. Their greatest gift is the ability to transform fear, hesitation, and doubt with the power of their compassion and love.

Distinguishing Features of Dancing Women

The most notable physical feature of the Dancing Woman is the shape of her long, narrow, thin lips. The distance between her Feathered Winged Serpent (clitoris) and the opening to her cave is nearly four fingers. This is the longest distance of all the anatomy types; the usual distance is two or three fingers or less from the clitoris to the vaginal opening.

Why Some Women Do Not Like Intercourse That Much

Additionally, a Dancing Woman's Fire Trigger is located very far back along the upper wall of her vaginal tunnel. It is actually beyond the reach of fingers, and in some cases even average-size tipilis. This makes it difficult (though not impossible) to simultaneously stimulate the ring of sensitive nerves at her opening, the clitoris, *and* her G-spot area through intercourse. This is the reason why, during typical penetration with fingers, or a tipili stroking inside, Dancing Women take a long time to climax. Dancing Woman may say that while intercourse is okay, it's not always all that great. They often need hands, or may use vibrators and dildos to stimulate their clitoris during intercourse. (This is also true for some of the other anatomy types.)

Pleasuring the Fire Trigger/G-Spot Area

Having a better understanding of where the G-spot area and the clitoris are located is extremely helpful to Dancing Women and their lovers. (See "Female Erogenous Zones of Pleasure" in chapter 6.) A Dancing Woman's pleasure increases greatly when she discovers that the clitoris and the entire inner cave are not only aroused through internal stroking—they are also stimulated externally. Because the Fire Trigger, or G-spot, branches in clusters of nerves within the spongy tissue underneath the Venus Mound (mons pubis), there is great erotic sensitivity on the outside of a woman's vulva too. Thus, one of the keys to delighting a Dancing Women is to use a lot of external grinding with a fair amount of pressure, different positions, and perhaps erotic toys along with either the hand or mouth. It's also why Dancing Women enjoy a lot of foreplay.

In my own experience listening to Dancing Women over the years, many are quite creative and determined to find the positions that really stimulate all their erotic zones of pleasure.

What One Dancing Woman Has to Say

After I found out I was a Dancing Woman, I felt truly relieved. First of all, it was embarrassing for me to always take so long to have an orgasm. A lot of times I would just give up because I felt like it was taking me way too long to come, and I was sure my husband was getting tired and probably bored too. It got to the point I was so frustrated I just shut down and pretty much avoided having sex. I felt like something was really wrong with me. Learning I am a Dancing Woman helps a lot because I don't feel like something is wrong, and it's nice to know other women have the same anatomy as I do.

Now I use a vibrator, or sometimes my husband reaches behind and touches my clit from behind while we are "spooning" for intercourse. We love the doggie position because if I arch my back, I can feel his penis touching my cervix. It used to take me about an hour to come, but since we have tried different positions and I'm not embarrassed to touch myself, it's a lot easier to have an orgasm. I think liking my "dancing" vagina more helps too.

DANCING WOMAN, MARY

Summary of Dancing Women

Direction on the Wheel: Center; catalyzes qualities in any direction

Distance Between Clitoris and Vaginal Opening: Three to four fingers average

Shape or Size of Hood: Small hood covers tiny clitoris that pops out easily

Inner Lips: Very narrow, thin, and long

Size of Cave/Entrance: Average, about five inches deep, $1\frac{1}{8}$" in diameter

Location of Fire Trigger (G-Spot Area): Very deep and back

Lubrication: Moist, damp

Temperature: Medium hot

Taste: Neutral

Typical Time to Reach Orgasm: Twenty to thirty minutes or longer

Types of Stimulation: Enjoys strong oral sex with sucking and side-to side flicking motion; sometimes enjoys direct clitoral stimulation; likes a lot of grinding with intercourse; often prefers additional stimulation with vibrator or fingers during intercourse (other types enjoy this as well)

Types of Orgasm: Varies

Preferred Intercourse Positions: May enjoy using a pillow under the small of the back to change the angle for penetration and allow thrusts to reach deeper; also enjoys legs together, doggie style, with a straight or arched back, along with manual stimulation

Preferred Male Anatomy Types: Enjoys Coyote Men because they like to grind the pubic mound; also likes Dancing Men and other types

Sexual Demeanor: Resourceful, spontaneous, intelligent, creative, and compassionate

9

Male Genital Anatomy Types

THE SACRED TIPILI

Knowing the many ways to arouse a man and finding out what he likes best is every bit as mysterious as discovering the secrets to a woman's pleasure. Just because a man has an erection and is ready to come does not mean he is anywhere near expressing his full sexual capacity. It is untrue that men are merely interested in ejaculating quickly. When given the invitation, they are eager to increase the intensity and duration of their sexual pleasure.

Although it's easier to see when they are aroused and when they are not, men yearn to experience the depth of their erotic natures. Learning a man's timing; the types of pressure, positions, and strokes he likes; and the sexual seductions that turn him on are the key ingredients to making his encounters especially good. While it is true that men are often happy with just about any sexual attention they are given, and they may not seem as particular as women, to satisfy a man's deeper desires you must know the details of his anatomy type. If you want to take a man into regions of sexual delight he rarely experiences, understanding his erotic temperament can significantly improve the quality of your lovemaking.

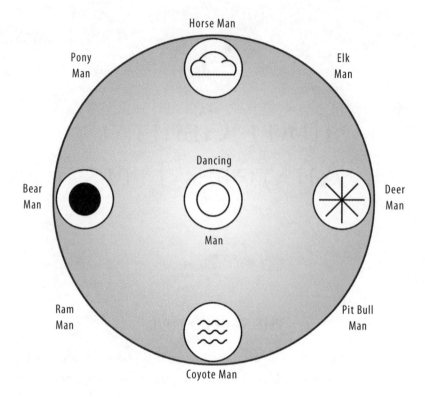

Fig. 9.1. Male Genital Anatomy Types

For men, there are fewer physical parts that make distinct differences in the way they reach orgasm. A man with a shorter penis, for instance, does not climax more quickly than a man with a larger one. Similarly, men with a larger glans do not enjoy oral sex more than men with smaller heads. Yet while the size of a man's tipili in no way changes the amount of pleasure he can experience, his genital anatomy does tell you what will intensify it the most. With practice, any man can become a better lover by learning to use his tipili with greater dexterity, especially if he also learns to use his hands, mouth, tongue, and mind with greater finesse. Knowing his genital anatomy type will give you insights into his weaknesses as well as his natural inclinations and creative abilities as a lover.[1]

HOW TO IDENTIFY A MAN'S
GENITAL ANATOMY TYPE

The simplest way to identify a man's genital anatomy type is by looking at the length and thickness of the erect tipili. In addition, the size and position of his testicles, the average number of ejaculation spurts, and the typical taste of his sexual secretions are used to determine his anatomy type.

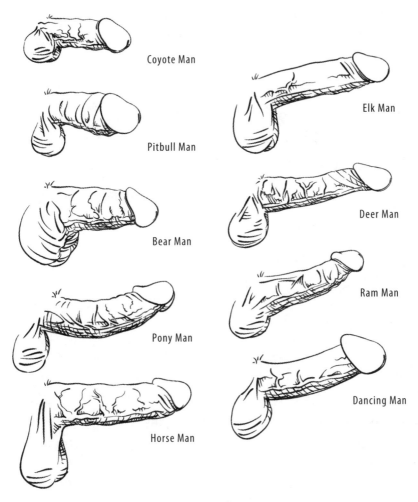

Fig. 9.2. Nine Male Anatomy Types

The Length

It is said that the average man's penis is twice the size of his thumb. Quodoushka measures the length of the male penis at full erection in terms of "hands." A hand means the measure across a man's open palm. The distance is measured from where the bottom of the index finger meets the palm, across the open hand to where the little finger meets the palm of the hand. (This distance is similar for all men and is measured by the man's own hands.) Thus, if a man places one palm face up with his little finger pressing against his body on the underside of his erect penis with the rest of his palm held flat underneath the shaft, he will either need to use one or two hands to measure his tipili.

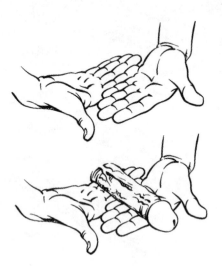

Fig. 9.3. Measuring Length

The Width

To measure the thickness—the width or girth—create a circle curling the thumb and first finger together and wrapping them around the erect tipili. You then count the joints where the tip of the first finger reaches the thumb. Thus for a tipili with a wide girth, the tip of the first finger may not reach the thumb, and with a narrower girth, the tip of the index finger will curl to meet the first or second joint along the inside of the thumb.

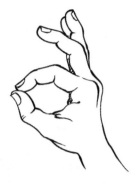

Fig. 9.4. Measuring Thickness

The Ejaculate

The tastes and amounts of ejaculate listed for each anatomy type describe men in a healthy state. Both men and women tend to have more profuse sexual secretions and reach orgasm more easily when they are highly aroused. As is the case with women, when a man is exhausted, stressed, or unhealthy, the amount, scent, and taste of his ejaculate can significantly change. The descriptions represent the usual taste of ejaculate as well as the average timing and amount of spurts.

Determining the Noncardinal Directions

Just as they are described for the female anatomy types, the noncardinal directions (Southwest, Northwest, Northeast, Southwest) for men have characteristics of the two adjacent cardinal directions. Thus, the tipili of an Elk Man (Northeast) is shorter than that of a Horse Man (North), and typically a bit thicker than that of a Deer Man (East). In addition, while he has a combination of both a Horse and a Deer Man's physical traits, his sexual temperament is also characterized by the attributes associated with those of an Elk Man.

ANATOMY PREFERENCES

As was mentioned for the female types, please keep in mind that physical anatomy does not limit sexual potential. With greater awareness, self-acceptance, and appreciation, when a Ram or Coyote Man (who has a shorter and narrower tipili than some of the other types) knows how to cultivate his sexual prowess, he can bring any woman to exceptional satis-faction. Likewise, when they hone their sensitivity, men with much larger tipilis can learn how to use size to their advantage. If you notice you have the physical attributes of a certain type, yet do not have all the sexual abilities described, it means you have a natural proclivity to develop these qualities.

Finally, remember that your anatomy is only a starting point, and that while you may have a preference for certain types, when you have the desire to know your lover well, you can be with anyone you choose.

SOUTH

Coyote Men

Coyote Men as Lovers

Coyotes are one of the most clever and resilient animals around. Their incredible ability to adapt and adjust to changing environments makes them one of the few species that can thrive close to humans in cities and towns. Native Americans call them tricksters because their cunning antics tend to get them in and out of all sorts of unusual situations.

Coyotes are notably intelligent, determined hunters. They cooperate and communicate with astute sophistication within the pack. They are also known for their playful natures and can often be seen chasing each other for fun in the middle of the day. As lovers, Coyote Men are the most resourceful, adaptable, and creative of all the genital anatomy types. They have kind hearts and are fun to be with. They are highly sexual, funny, mischievous, and most of all persistent.

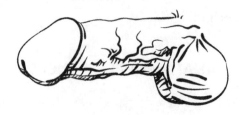

Fig. 9.5. Coyote Man

When hunting, coyotes shift their techniques in accordance with their prey. Using their keen sense of smell to track down what they want, they slowly close in, circle through the grass, and when ready to pounce, they stiffen in a catlike manner. Like the coyote, Coyote Men pursue sexual partners with great diligence and resolve, often for years. They can be courageous in the face of rejection and have an unusual ability to tune in to a woman's emotional needs and desires. They listen well, adjust their techniques, and then shift their approach to please. They can be disarmingly charming when they use humor and laughter to seduce during courtship and foreplay. They love giving (and receiving) oral sex.

When they go too far, however, and are too determined to get what they want, they come off as being overly clingy. Coyote Men need to acquire a set of sexual skills by becoming masters of oral sex, using their hands, and getting good at the special grinding motion with their hips that many women love. Their biggest challenge is to gain self-confidence, particularly with regard to the size of their tipilis. They need to turn their size into an asset by understanding that women feel the energy of the cock as much as its physical size. This means women feel the force of the ejaculate along with the dexterity of the penis. Coyote Men can learn to touch various places inside the vagina with precision and care and have the capacity to feel many more subtle sensations in their tipilis than men with larger members. Furthermore, because a Coyote Man sits in the South of the wheel, he has the ability to soothe a woman's emotions with the thrust of his pure heart. Once he has the confidence to use his powerful sensitivity, he can enhance intercourse with the erotic foreplay many women enjoy. At their best, Coyote Men are selfless givers. Their instinctive drive to take women to multiple peaks of pleasure is beyond compare.

Distinguishing Features of Coyote Men

One of the notable features of Coyote Men is the short length and narrow girth of their tipilis. When a Coyote Man takes his persistent nature and uses it to become skilled with his mouth and hands as well as his tipili, he can bring any partner to ecstatic bliss. Coyote Men should realize that women enjoy all these ways of lovemaking.

Summary of Coyote Men

Direction on the Wheel: South, the place of emotions and water and giving

Length of Shaft: One hand and a head or less (this means the shaft reaches across the palm and the head extends slightly further than one hand)

Thickness: Index finger to first joint of thumb or less

Loads or Spurts of Ejaculate: Typical number of spurts is six to twelve

Timing: Fast, rapid fire

Temperature: Hot

Taste of Ejaculate: Sweet

Consistency of Ejaculate: Watery, thin

Position of Testicles: Fit fairly close to the body

Temperament and Demeanor: Resourceful, resilient, persistent, humorous, and sensuously receptive

SOUTHWEST

Pit Bull (Dog) Men

Pit Bull (Dog) Men as Lovers

Because dogs are one of the most domesticated animals on the planet and have lived intimately with humans for thousands of years, they have developed a variety of distinct personalities. They have strong bodies and sense danger the instant it appears. The pit bull has a tenacious willingness to serve and is wired to protect its companions with unstoppable zeal. As lovers, Pit Bull Men urgently desire to give their lovers the pleasure they desire.

All dogs respond to the way they are treated in their home environments. They are as sensitive to tension and stress as they are to passion and play. The simple rule for being with Pit Bull Men is to give what you most desire to receive. Approach them calmly if you wish them to be peaceful,

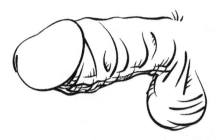

Fig. 9.6. Pit Bull Man

and approach them with passion if you want excitement and fun. Above all, for Pit Bull Men to express their full sexual potential, they need to establish their place, know their territory, and trust their partners. When they receive clear, consistent messages and feel genuinely wanted, these men are loyal for life. Some Pit Bull Men are loners; others crave a great deal of affection and dislike being left out; while others are rambunctious and flirtatious. It all depends on the kind of attention they get from their lovers.

Pit Bull Men require partners who treat them respectfully with a firm hand and stable boundaries. They like having rules to follow and a clear understanding of their responsibilities as partners. Chaos causes them to feel insecure, and disorder triggers their aggression. It is thus very important to provide clear, uncomplicated signals with a Pit Bull Man. At the same time, they are great explorers. They have a hunger to try new things—from the most kinky to the most romantic seductions; they will forever surprise you with with their relentless pursuit of pleasure.

While it is often a challenge for these men to plainly share their sexual needs and desires, they yearn to be heard and understood. Pit Bull Men must learn to lighten up, be less jealous, and let go of placing strong demands on their lovers. They need to discover and master what they are naturally good at without looking for immediate rewards. When they subdue their aggression by doing things they love, their passion and loyalty is unsurpassed. To charm and arouse a Pit Bull Man, give him unambiguous signals that you truly want him. If you welcome him into your bed by your warmth and affection, he'll wag his tail and return your favors a thousandfold.

Distinguishing Features of Pit Bull Men

Physically, a Pit Bull's tipili is longer than a Coyote's and nearly as thick as a Bear's. He is known for his steady climb to climax and his intensely faithful attention to his lover's pleasure. He is exceptionally fond of making sure his partner is more than satisfied.

Summary of Pit Bull Men

Direction on the Wheel: Southwest, the place of dreams, symbols, and exploration

Physical Anatomy: Tipili is longer than a Coyote Man's, almost as thick as a Bear Man's

Temperament and Demeanor: Tenaciously loyal, powerful, full of life, adventurous, and friendly

WEST

Bear Men

Bear Men as Lovers

Except when they are courting, bears are typically solitary animals. Of all the male types, the Bear Man is the most physically present; he likes to hug, hold, and cuddle his partner during lovemaking. Bear Men can be stocky, strong, and at times lumbering and slow, yet when the heat of passion rises, Bear Men are stunningly swift and strong. The potent

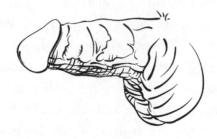

Fig. 9.7. Bear Man

charge of their loving thrusts can carry their lovers deep into the mystery and magic of sexual trance. Bear Men have an affinity for finding lifelong friendships and love.

Bear Men truly cherish the physical feelings of connected intimacy. They thrive by having a steady source of warm feminine energy and like the comforts of a home and hearth. They are gifted with natural sexual prowess and sometimes like to fall asleep inside their partner, dreaming through the night after making love. When Bear Men bond sexually, they will safeguard loved ones with fierce courage. They thus make dependable, devoted partners who yearn for the joys of enduring companionship. Charming and courting a Bear Man is easy. He seeks true friendship and responds to steadfast, unwavering affection. He needs to know you are there to stay.

Bear Men are, however, prone to loneliness and get needy when they don't get the attention they crave. Bears regularly retreat into their caves for winter sleep to recharge themselves, and thus their medicine is the keeper of dreams. Bear Men can be visionary leaders. They can take their partners deep into healing dream states and provide security and support for their daily dreams as well.

Bears often lay down false tracks and are notorious for doubling back on anything tracking them. They are extremely clever, and it's impossible to predict what they will do. This is actually one of the things that make Bear Men so attractive: they can be capricious, impulsive, and whimsical. When they are happy, they go out of their way to give special things and love to surprise their partners with affectionate gifts. They may disappear from time to time, but they will return to share insights from their solitary journeys.[2]

Because they tend to retreat into their own worlds and lapse into long periods of brooding uncertainty, Bear Men need to communicate their sexual desires with clarity and conviction. They can be slow, patient, and overly defensive and thus seem to take forever, doing only things they want to do. For a Bear Man to manifest the gifts he hopes to offer, he needs to overcome his moody hesitations and take decisive actions that spring from the passion of his heart. When Bear Men conquer their fears of being vulnerable and weak and learn to express their needs for intimacy and sexual love, their optimism overflows with commanding authority. Strengthened with a steadfast source of feminine intimacy, a Bear Man will not only face any obstacle to protect what is meaningful to him, he will courageously care for the fragile aspirations of his lovers and maintain unbending bonds of freedom and trust.

Distinguishing Features of Bear Men

Bear Men's tipilis are very thick and fairly long, although not as long as a Pony or Horse Man's. Their testicles are fairly small and compact, and when they are aroused they draw back tightly toward the groin area. Usually, a Bear Man's semen has a somewhat Clorox-like odor, which becomes more astringent if he is unhealthy or stressed. While all men's semen will change in scent if they are unhealthy, this is particularly true for Bear Men.

Summary of Bear Men

Direction on the Wheel: West, place of the body, Earth, holding and transforming with intimacy

Length of Shaft: One to two hands

Thickness: Thick, two to four inches in diameter

Loads of Spurts of Ejaculate: One to two spurts with pauses in between

Timing: Slow

Temperature: Cool

Taste of Ejaculate: Sweet-sour, sharp taste (like Clorox or astringent if imbalanced)

Consistency of Ejaculate: Thick, white, honeylike

Position of Testicles: Tight and close to the body

Temperament and Demeanor: Intensely affectionate, supportive, protective, courageous, visionary dreamers

NORTHWEST

Pony Men

Pony Men as Lovers

Ponies bear many of the powerful qualities of horses; they are considered smart and friendly, though sometimes are known to be stubborn. Pony Men have lighthearted, fun-loving, and generous natures. They are fond of intelligent women and are stimulated by lively, spirited conversation. Pony Men bring a lot of humor and use playful gestures to show their eagerness in the bedroom. They are endowed with incredibly persistent, gentle strength as lovers, and they love being mounted and taken for a good ride. Like Horse Men, they have an innate sense of justice and will frequently go out of their way to help others in need—sometimes forgetting their own responsibilities in the process.

Like Bear Men, they also need definite and sometimes extended periods of alone time. However, not only do Pony Men recharge their creative energy with solitude and dreamy reverie, they are also highly social creatures. They like to rove freely, traveling around to see the sights. If they use these times of freedom wisely, Pony Men return to their lovers eager to share their adventures. Their robust enthusiasm for life frequently makes them magnets for wealth, friendships, and dynamic relationships.

Pony Men need to be careful they do not become stubbornly tied in to their emotional fears and insecurities. If they feel trapped or cornered, they will bite back in fits of anger, and if they feel insecure about their sexual

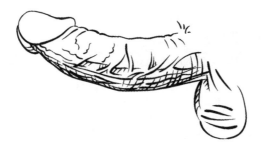

Fig. 9.8. Pony Man

performance, they will shrink with doubt. They can also be deviously determined to get what they want. When Ponies learn to allow their lovers the freedom to discover the independence they themselves desire, and rein in their fears of being left alone, they become feisty, energetic, and faithful partners. Above all, Pony Men yearn to yield in the arms of strong, loving feminine beauty. They thrive when they have plenty of interesting pursuits to get into and don't have to hold back their sexual power. If given the freedom to disappear from time to time, along with plenty of praise when they return, Pony Men will shower their partners with sincere gratitude. While they may not always show it, they are secretly romantic lovers.

Distinguishing Features of Pony Men

Pony Men have the girth of Bear Men and Horse Men. It can take a whole hand to grasp a Pony Man's shaft fully, and sometimes a woman's fingers will not meet with her thumb around his erect tipili. A Pony's length is greater than that of a Bear Man, yet shorter than that of a Horse. His testicles do not hang as low as a Horse Man's and are somewhat more closely pulled into his body. Some Pony Men may take a long time to become hard, or may at times have difficulty ejaculating. While this can also happen for other anatomy types, delayed ejaculations occur more frequently for Pony and Horse Men. When these men feel their partner is enjoying giving them pleasure, and know they have all the time in the world, these difficulties subside. As Pony Men relax into their easygoing natures and let go of any sexual goals, their sexual potency stays steady and strong.

Summary of Pony Men

Direction on the Wheel: Northwest; the place of pattern, timing, and Sacred Body Image

Physical Anatomy: Between Horse and Bear; almost as long as a Horse Man, has the thickness of a Bear Man

Temperament and Demeanor: Determined, feisty, charming, alternately compliant and strong willed with powerful sex drives

NORTH

Horse Man

Horse Men as Lovers

Horse Men exude a sense of pride and confidence in their stride. Horses are poised long-distance runners who love following their partner's commands. In the Sweet Medicine teachings, the horse is the carrier of the beliefs of the people because of its ability to connect, understand, and communicate well with humans. Horse Men are great companions, and they are as drawn to a woman's mental prowess as they are to her physical beauty.

Because they are so intelligent and enjoy the game of learning their lover's sensuous secrets, they can become highly responsive connoisseurs of love and sex. Like Pony Men, they are obstinate at times and spooked by surprises. They shy away from harshness and dislike being overly controlled. However, if you whisper in a Horse Man's ear, and you gently lead him, you can take him anywhere you want to go. Horse Men like being seduced, and they love to gallop.

Horse Men yearn to share their considerable talents with the world and have an easy time meeting, attracting, and satisfying lovers, yet they can be too sure of themselves in the bedroom. Some Horse Men are like "hotblooded" racehorses—energetic, sensitive, and fast. Others are like "coldblooded" draft horses—steady, quiet, and secure. At times Horse Men are content to graze in the pastures and are happy to stay close to home, but they need to run wild from time to time. Once a Horse

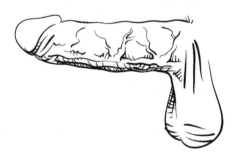

Fig. 9.9. Horse Man

Man feels needed and desired, he will take you the heights and valleys of extreme passion and show you the powerhouse of joy he yearns to give.

Horse Men need to be careful about building resentments and feeling saddled down by too many responsibilities. When they take on the challenge of commitments they want to make, and have the time to make their far-reaching ideas happen, their sexual relationships flourish. As a Horse Man turns his intelligence inward and develops the intuition to know when to lead and when to follow, his true power emerges. In fact, for a Horse Man to become a thoroughbred lover, he needs to align closely with the wisest source of divine feminine energy he can find. When he does, a Horse Man becomes one of the most reliable, committed, and trustworthy partners of all the anatomy types.

Distinguishing Features of Horse Men

Often regarded as stallions or studs, Horse Men are recognized by the unusual length and girth of their tipilis. Their testicles are also large and hang low. Over the years I have met many Horse Men who face a number of sexual challenges. Rather than always being regarded as superior lovers, they tell me many women are afraid they won't be able to handle their large size. Thus some Horse Men who have had this type of rejection repress their innate sexual power for fear of hurting the woman they are with. However, any Horse Man can learn to slow his pace and become better skilled at finding the timing, sufficient lubrication, and positions to ensure his partners' comfort and pleasure.

In addition, while many Horse Men can sustain hours of intense sexual play, they have a hard time accepting that they cannot always maintain their erections for as long as they would like. When they feel they cannot perform to their own high standards, Horse Men (and other types as well) avoid opportunities for intimate connection. It can be quite a challenge for a Horse Man to develop the qualities he needs as a lover, in part because he may think he knows what women want. For any man, but especially the Horse Man, the more he asks questions, lets go of his pride, and shows his vulnerability, the more his strength can shine.

Summary of Horse Men

Direction on the Wheel: North, the place of the mind, wind, and receiving with care

Length of Shaft: Two hands and a head or longer

Thickness: Two to four inches or more

Amounts of Ejaculate: Typical number of spurts: eight to ten, profuse

Timing: Fairly slow

Temperature: Warm

Taste of Ejaculate: Semisweet to salty

Consistency of Ejaculate: Medium thick, milky white

Position of Testicles: Large, sometimes hanging low

Temperament and Demeanor: Intelligent, intense stamina and endurance, confident, alternately yielding and strong willed

NORTHEAST

Elk Men

Elk Men as Lovers

The elk is one of the largest and most majestic animals of the forest. Thunder Strikes tells a story about an elk he encountered while hunting as a young man.

"By mid-afternoon the storm broke with intense thunder, lightning, and downpour. I caught sight of a big buck elk standing on a high ridge not far away. I stopped in my tracks as I saw the jagged lightning strike his antlers and his whole body take on a glow. The elk stood there, absorbing the full charge of the lightning. Then I watched him calmly dip his antlers into the stream."

He ran home to tell his teachers about the "magic elk" he thought he'd seen. They split their guts laughing. "It wasn't a magic elk," they

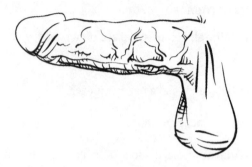

Fig. 9.10. Elk Man

explained, "The elk is the keeper of thunder and lightning and a master choreographer of energy." It is said that years later, Stella Many Names, a matriarch of the Twisted Hairs Council of Elders, pointed out, "When you are given the gift of a Sweet Medicine teaching (or see an animal in its moment of power), you can approach it in its space or territory. If you would have stayed and approached the elk, it would have taught you how it transformed lightning."[3] As lovers, Elk Men have the capacity to transform the "lightning" of their seeds, including both their thoughts and ejaculations, into explosive moments of power. Like the mature bull that will defend his harem of cows from competitors with his thunderous bellows, Elk Men are not afraid to fight for someone they love. They have the capacity to absorb negative energy and redirect it for healing. They are sturdy, energetic, but sometimes paradoxical partners who rarely do the expected.[4]

Elk Men yearn to find a companion who wants what they have to offer and who can help direct their power and courage into focused outcomes. Elk Men are drawn to help others, and they are particularly susceptible to rescuing damsels in distress. Their challenge is to bring their visions down to Earth, subdue their restlessness, and be more sexually creative. To charm and arouse an Elk Man, treat his accomplishments as magical expressions of his love and care. Welcome him into an inviting, warm hearth along with plenty of sex and space to be himself, and he will build a kingdom filled with lovingkindness.

Distinguishing Features of Elk Men

Elk Men are characterized physically by having a long tipili, slightly longer than that of a Deer Man, and less thick than that of a Horse Man. An Elk Man's tipili frequently has a natural "tilt" toward the left or right. Sexually, their pace is sometimes quick, sometimes slow, and they reach the peak of arousal by varying the timing of their thrusts. They truly enjoy riding on the edge of sexual pleasure and enjoy being teased to climax. Sexually, they can surprise you with their lightening speed. They have a distinctive way of being able to coax their lovers to go for more by transforming their shyness and resistance into open, uninhibited releases of blissful rapture.

Summary of Elk Men

Direction on the Wheel: Northeast; place of focus, relaxation, and design of energy

Physical Anatomy: Between the length of a Horse Man and a Deer Man, narrower than a Horse Man, thicker than a Deer Man; shaft often angles slightly to the left or right

Temperament and Demeanor: Charismatic leaders, mysterious and magical transformers, kindhearted, persuasive energy designers

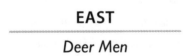

EAST

Deer Men

Deer Men as Lovers

Noted for being quick and alert, deer are regarded as being the most graceful of all the forest animals. They have lithe, compact bodies with long, powerful legs suited for rugged terrain. Like the deer, Deer Men are some of the most attractive and alluring of all the male anatomy types. They have exceptional stamina and stunning quickness, and are supremely alert to women's sexual desires. They are naturally seductive, charismatic, and extremely passionate partners.

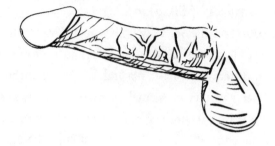

Fig. 9.11. Deer Man

Yaqui Indians have practiced the Deer Dance for hundreds of years, emulating the deer's elegant magical powers. Their dance reflects the deer's ability to be in a constant state of harmony and balance within chaos. As they enact the mating ritual where bucks fight for the right to attract females, the males bow their antlers, circle one another, bend back their hind legs, lower their heads, and charge. This nicely describes the magical sexual temperament of Deer Men.

Indigenous deer can live in many kinds of environments. They are selective feeders that roam and browse for just the right food. Deer Men are similarly discerning and are constantly on the lookout for unusual sexual experiences. They are good at creating several sexual possibilities at once. Deer Men sit in the East of the wheel, the place of fire and spirit. They posses expansive, magnanimous spirits and have a magnetic quality. They are warm, generous, and powerfully explosive lovers who have the inherent ability to release their creative ideas with compelling élan. They share insights and feelings beautifully and have an uncanny way of knowing precisely how to melt away a woman's defenses.

To charm and court a Deer Man, you should take him into places where he cannot go by himself. Although he seems elusive sometimes and likes to dazzle you with his brilliance, he yearns to look more deeply into himself. Like all men, he needs to feel loved and appreciated for who he is. Because they are such naturally gifted seducers, Deer Men can easily become overconfident to the point where their charms become a turn-off. They must accept more meaningful challenges instead of going for easy game. To avoid becoming too arrogant and proud, they need to be less self-centered in their giving. When they make abiding commitments and satisfy their hunger for highly charged sexual encounters, Deer Men can focus their artistic imagination and make astonishing contributions to the world.

Distinguishing Features of Deer Men

A Deer Man has a long, narrow tipili that is often tapered at the end. Typically, his testicles hang very low, and often one is much lower than the other. Sexually, he is fond of prolonged, penetrating, and deep-thrusting sensual love. Deer Men can be unusually romantic lovers whose passion drives them to become skilled in the intricacies of loving touch. Deer Men have the potential to become artisans in the secrets of carnal desire.

Summary of Deer Men

Direction on the Wheel: East; fire, spirit, determining with passion and lust

Length of Shaft: Two hands and a head

Thickness: Index finger to the thumb's tip or to the first joint of the thumb

Amounts of Ejaculate: Three to six

Timing: Fast

Temperature: Hot

Taste of Ejaculate: Slightly tart, very salty

Consistency of Ejaculate: Milky thin

Position of Testicles: One testicle usually hangs lower then the other

Temperament and Demeanor: Alluringly seductive, charming, and powerfully magnetic lovers

SOUTHEAST

Ram Men

Ram Men as Lovers

Rams are rugged, agile rock climbers that fearlessly scale the heights and like to wander in the open air. Young mountain goats are incredibly feisty players that love to test their strength and prowess by playing king of the mountain.[5] Unlike sheep who follow the leader, rams do not abide by the strict hierarchies of herds. In Greek mythology the story of the Golden Fleece describes the ram's unstoppable quest to find his legitimacy and become king. Men with this genital anatomy type are true seekers who are not easily crushed by rejections or failures. Their powerful sex drives are charged with great tenacity because the pursuit of the hunt turns them on.

As lovers, Ram Men are energetic, vigorous, and highly erotic. Their passion comes out in fast, powerful bursts, and they are not afraid to go into the deeply mysterious places of sexual love. At home they are somewhat stoic, preferring to keep things to themselves. Intimate conversation does not come easily to a Ram, and he rarely speaks his mind directly to his partner. However, his playful humor and youthful demeanor comes out in social groups, making him the center of attraction. Ram Men are fearlessly flirtatious and love to test their sexual wiles. They are action oriented. When they are being adored and accepted, they become irresistibly alluring. They have the spirit and charisma of a Deer Man along with the sensitivity and persistence of a Coyote Man.

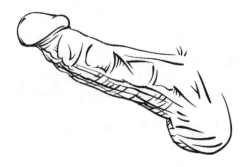

Fig. 9.12. Ram Man

According to Chinese astrology, those born in the Year of the Ram have a tendency to be impractical or careless with money, and they have a tendency to meander and procrastinate. Ram Men can become sacrificial lambs when they retreat into their doubts and insecurities. They are also prone to butting heads and duels of strength where they waste too much energy posturing for a superior position. When Ram Men learn to express their needs directly and assert their strength without masked aggression, they bring tremendous vitality to their lovers. Most of all, rather than burning out in quick blasts, these men must pace themselves in love and sex and they must learn to become more committed lovers willing to go through the ups and downs of relationships.

To court and arouse a Ram, treat him like a king by giving him genuine praise. If you treat him with respect and dignity, he will shower you with vitality and take you into the hidden mysteries of sexual love.

Distinguishing Features of Ram Men

Ram Men are easily roused to erection, and their tipilis frequently project upward at a 45-degree angle. Their tipilis are narrow like the Deer Man's and longer than the Coyote Man's. When they are near climax their thrusts become fast and furious, something like a battering ram. As partners, Ram Men are fun-loving teasers and can be uniquely naughty lovers who are strengthened by the challenge of being with enthusiastic, independent women.

Summary of Ram Men

Direction on the Wheel: Southeast; self-love, self-concepts, attitude, and approach

Physical Anatomy: Between Coyote Man and Deer Man

Temperament and Demeanor: Agile, energetic, youthful, proud and fearless lovers

CENTER

Dancing Man

Dancing Men as Lovers

Because Dancing Men sit in the middle of the Medicine Wheel, they alternately express attributes of each direction. They are known as the great transformers of energy because they can change their approach from one moment to the next. Dancing Men can be the most sensitive of all the anatomy types to the fluctuations of a woman's desires. They have the ability to listen beyond words, tune into the body's erotic language, and give their lovers what they really need. Like Deer Women, they love reaching into the magical, mysterious spaces of sensuously carnal delight.

Dancing Men often treat their lovers with trust and honesty and are willing to communicate with open hearts. They like learning different techniques and are eager to step outside their routines to find more creative sexual things to do. Dancing Men live to uncover new ways to satisfy and enchant their lovers. They are diligent seekers of pleasure and knowledge. Their seeds are like multifaceted arrows searching for ways to join with feminine energy in beauty.

At times they can be as persistent and resourceful as Coyote Men. They can be as feisty and loyal as a Pit Bull or as cuddly as a Bear Man. They are as powerful as Pony Men and can have the endurance of Horse Men. If the moment calls, they will turn on their charisma like a Deer

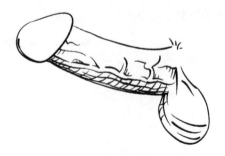

Fig. 9.13. Dancing Man

Man, be as mysterious as an Elk Man, and become as agile and playful as a Ram Man.

Once they have chosen a direction, their greatest challenge is to stay on course without becoming inflexible. Dancing Men can be fickle and impatient. They meander and are often stressed, wondering whether they are going in the right direction. Especially with affairs of the heart, they hesitate around the wheel, trying to make the perfect decision before they act. When Dancing Men avoid the temptation to escape conflict, dare to boldly pursue what they want, take a stand, and then act decisively. They gain the fulfillment that comes from enjoying the small pleasures of mundane affairs. If you want to court and arouse a Dancing Man, let him know he is special and that you trust his decisions. Assure him that his explorations and achievements are worthy, and then keep him on his toes with unexpected erotic surprises.

Distinguishing Features of Dancing Men

Dancing Men have average-sized tipilis with tapered heads. They are the most common of the male anatomy types. They enjoy all kinds of women and can become masterful lovers because they are willing to use their hands, their body, vibrators, oral sex, or whatever it takes to bring their partner into the highest states of pleasure possible. They enjoy just about every position imaginable. The uniqueness of the Dancing Man lies in his natural humility, which comes from his unassuming, nonboastful manner. One of his most attractive qualities is the way he makes his lovers feel at ease by accepting and embracing their vulnerabilities and encouraging them to shine.

Summary of Dancing Men

Direction on the Wheel: Center, the void, the energy that catalyzes the entire wheel with open heart-to-heart communication

Length of Shaft: Two hands

Thickness: Index finger to last joint of thumb tip

Loads or Spurts of Ejaculate: Four to eight

Timing: Fast

Temperature: Medium warm

Taste of Ejaculate: Salty

Consistency of Ejaculate: Creamy

Testicles: Average size

Temperament and Demeanor: Accommodating, dexterous, creative, and charming explorers who are willing and hungry to learn

10

THE Nine Types OF Orgasmic Expression

Our bodies know which type of orgasm we need most. Our main job is to let go of the pretender voices that inhibit us from expressing our natural sexual feelings. Orgasms make us feel lighter and happier; they can heal wounds, help us feel whole, and reconnect us with all of life.

AN EXPANDED VIEW OF ORGASMS

We commonly think of an orgasm as the culmination of intense genital pleasure accompanied by involuntary convulsions and euphoric feelings. Quodoushka extends this meaning to include the entire spectrum of physical and emotional expressions within any sexual experience. Inspired by observing the great universal forces of nature, the Wheel of Orgasmic Expression teaches about the potential power of orgasms to restore balance in the physical body. Orgasms allow the mind to stretch beyond usual consciousness, nourish our bodies, and fill the spirit with truth and beauty.

Viewed this way, an orgasm becomes something much more than a mere energy boost. An expanded view of orgasm includes every sensation from those tiny pleasant shudders traveling up our spines to the powerful rolling bolts of electricity that draw our bodies close, and that cause our spirits to merge together in cosmic union. These great energy waves transport our ordinary awareness and make us feel peaceful and whole. Understanding that we have different types of orgasms—from small sparks to grand explosions—prevents us from being disappointed when we do not experience the big bang we think we ought to have every time.

In Malaysia many years ago, a young woman approached me after a talk I gave on the beauty and power of sex. She lived in a conservative Muslim, Hindu, and Christian society, and it was the first time she had heard someone speak publicly about sex. When we left the lecture hall, she came over to ask, "Are you saying those trembles I feel are orgasms? I've had sex, but I'm not really sure if I've ever had an orgasm." I remember the look of relief on her face when I told her, "Yes. Those feelings are mini-orgasms. If you enjoy them like small coals, and let them get hotter, sooner or later those trembles will erupt like a volcano inside you."

Since then, many men and women have asked similar questions about what can be considered an orgasm. Because we generally expect an intense explosion, we discount many of the more subtle sensations happening along the way. Holding an image in our minds of what our bodies should do limits the healing power of our full orgasmic expression. Over time, truncating the potency and duration of subtle sensations weakens our libido and causes us to have lower-level orgasms. It's not merely whether we have "had an orgasm," rather we should ask, have we expressed ourselves fully?

As you will see from the descriptions of various types of orgasms, even the shivers you feel while watching a beautiful sunset can be included in your orgasmic repertoire. Of course it feels great to explode with energy, but if you are having difficulty reaching those peaks, start with enjoying the feelings you have.

ORGASMS ARE A SIGN OF WHAT WE NEED

One of the reasons we enjoy orgasms so much is that while certain parts of our brains are lighting up and others are shutting down, and those feel-good hormones are rushing through the bloodstream, we get a respite from everyday thinking. For a brief time, we can hear, see, feel, and even taste things more clearly. Our best orgasms are spontaneous, and each one shows us just what our bodies need. Some orgasms take us into quiet moments of inner solace; some leave us doubled over in uncontrollable laughter; while others send our minds into another time and dimension. They make us cry, sing, bond, or quake with pleasure. Each of these expressions helps us reach a state of equilibrium, vitality, and peace.

Describing orgasms on a wheel makes each direction equal; none has any higher place than any other. A South orgasm balances emotions by releasing laughter or tears; a West orgasm restores the body with powerful shakes and tremors. North orgasms come in gusts that clear the mind, and East orgasms ignite our creative spirits.

DIFFERENT STROKES FOR DIFFERENT FOLKS

Many recent books seek to help people have better sex. You can find videos on the G-spot, ejaculation, and multiple orgasms. You can learn to have five-minute quickies or hours of extended play. Quodoushka celebrates exploring a wide range of sexual expression and goes further to explain how the types and levels of orgasms restore health. Instead of describing female orgasms solely by the place they originate (a clitoral or a vaginal orgasm), it explains how orgasms for women either implode or explode. For example, when a woman curls into a fetal position, the energy of her orgasm is pulling her inward, whereas when she arches back in climax, her orgasm is explosive and outward. Implosive orgasms help us become more open, intuitive, and receptive, explosive expressions expand our ability to act creatively.

For a man, different types of orgasms are described in part by whether he has an erect, semi-erect, or flaccid penis. One comes with no erection and a full ejaculation of fluid, while others are marked by energy releases alone. Some orgasms focus intensely in the genitals, while others do not. Most men mistakenly narrow their sexual expression to one image: a hard erection with a full ejaculation of semen. Although this highly pleasurable orgasm is greatly favored, and it is deeply satisfying, other expressions can be equally fulfilling. It should also be noted that orgasm is not synonymous with ejaculation; they are two important but distinct functions within our orgasmic expressions.

Early Ejaculation

Quodoushka teaches that except in the case of severe physical disorders, chronic early ejaculation is entirely preventable. Every man is likely, at some point in his life, to feel insecure about coming too early or not being able to satisfy his partner. The male orgasm wheel goes a long way toward helping us more fully understand what is happening during a man's orgasm. Emotions are commonly associated with female sexuality, but men also have various emotional responses that generate different kinds of orgasms.

For example, when a man learns that having a South Avalanche Orgasm (with a soft or semi-erect penis and a full ejaculation of fluids) is brought on by deep feelings for his partner, he can learn to relax and be more intimate during times his tipili is semi-hard. Rather than pulling away, considering his response premature, he can stay connected and enjoy the special healing powers of the South orgasm.

When men value the full range of their orgiastic expressions, instead of losing energy and worrying about performance, they can embrace the natural cycles of their sexual rhythms. By accepting all our sexual expressions, we can improve the quality of our lovemaking and become more compassionate, caring lovers. The Heart-Pleasuring Exercise explained in chapter 12 will increase the intensity of every type of orgasm.

For both men and women, each orgasmic expression brings the gift of one of the five Huaquas. As stated earlier, when we have a "South" orgasm, it gives us the gift of Happiness, the West generates Health, the North brings us Humor, the East brings Hope, and Center orgasms bring the gift of Harmony.

MALE ORGASMS

HAWK
FULL ERECTION, NO EJACULATION
WITH FULL ORGASM
Wind orgasm, gusts of wind in bursts. Focus in mind
and genitals. When you feel almost at the point of no
return, relax all muscles, especially the buttocks and
take rhythmic breaths to kick you into orgasm.
TORNADO

CROW/RAVEN
FULL ERECTION,
FULL EJACULATION
WITH FULL ORGASM
Earth orgasm, body
sweeping chills and
shudders. Whole body
quakes, genital focus.
EARTHQUAKE

**THUNDERBIRD/
PHOENIX**
Total body orgasm,
fire breath orgasm,
catalyst to experiencing
the whole wheel.

EAGLE
NO ERECTION,
NO EJACULATION,
WITH FULL ORGASM
Fire orgasm, heat waves
rising up from genitals and
spreading through entire
body. Genital focus while
body feels like it is on fire.
RAGING FOREST FIRE

OWL
PARTIAL ERECTION, NO ERECTION
FULL EJACULATION, WITH FULL ORGASM
Water orgasm, comes in slow waves, heart
and emotion focus. Can be overwhelming
emotional passion.
AVALANCHE

Fig. 10.1. Male Orgasm Expression

SOUTH

Avalanche Orgasm

*I remember when I was a young man, I was infatuated
by this girl at college. I thought about her all the time,
and in fact she was my first "love." I finally mustered the
courage to ask her out to a party. By the time we came
back to my dorm room, I was so excited I thought I was*

going to explode. We made out on the desk, and everything
was incredible. But I had been waiting almost a year for
this moment. By the time she unzipped my pants and
kissed me, well, that was it, or so I thought back then. I
was devastated. If I could rewind the clock and just realize
what was happening, I could have saved myself so much
anguish.

BRUCE, AGE THIRTY-TWO

The Avalanche Orgasm is a South, water expression. It starts to build up slowly and comes in gradual waves of intensity. Because there is so much focus on the emotions and heart, the tipili may not be hard. There may be a partial erection or no erection. The buildup is followed by a full, usually unexpected, ejaculation and orgasm. Often, premature or early ejaculation happens because of overwhelming passion. Fortunately, any man can learn to enjoy and relax into the powerful sensations in his flaccid penis. It does not mean he is not turned on. On the contrary, it usually means he is flooded with feelings.

South Avalanche Orgasms may become more frequent after a man turns sixty. If he accepts the changes of his body, and can move into the feelings that occur during this type of orgasm, his sensations will be deeper and his ejaculations will feel very intense. Even self-pleasuring with a semi-erect or flaccid tipili can be extremely satisfying and it can become a rejuvenating solution for so-called impotence.

If an early ejaculation does occur the best thing to do is to just let it happen. Try to let go of the idea that the only thing that matters is an extremely hard tipili. The truth is, many women love the texture and feeling of a man's genitals when they are in this softer state, especially for oral sex. If partners take their time, stay intimate, and rejoice in the pleasurable connection, then other types of orgasms on the wheel are possible. Frequently, men who enjoy these feelings (rather than thinking it's over) are able to take their passion into extended sexual play. This is where a little bit of patience, and even laughter, goes a long way.

Avalanche Expression

Think of falling snow on a huge mountain. The snow keeps falling and falling on an overhang until finally, one more flake of falling snow is just too much. The whole cliff cascades downward and comes crashing down in full force.

Owl Expression

The owl is a silent predator of the night. It glides effortlessly in flight until in one surprising moment it sees its prey. With no warning, in a quick instant, the unsuspecting creature must surrender. This is the energy of the Owl Expression, which approaches quietly and happens suddenly. The gift of the Avalanche/Owl Orgasm is to allow the more nuanced and delicate sensations of love to be shared. Vulnerability and softness are two of nature's greatest and most powerful attributes. South orgasms give us the "Huaqua" or the gift of Happiness.

NORTH

Tornado Orgasm

I didn't realize I could stay hard so long without ever ejaculating. At first I tried switching positions, and then I tried having oral sex. But nothing worked, and I couldn't come like I usually do. This went on and on until it finally dawned on me that I actually felt really good. After that, we made love all afternoon, and it didn't matter to me anymore that I wasn't coming. A couple of times though it really felt like I did.

JOHN, AGE FORTY-ONE

This orgasm is a North, wind expression. It comes in strong, intermittent bursts of energetic surges with a high stimulating charge. Partners are engaged with a mental and genital focus. A wind orgasm can be generated by lots of conversation, fantasy, or erotic talk. The man's tipili is in full erection, often for an extended period. At the peak of climax he has a full orgasm with no fluid ejaculation. Sometimes, men who experience this type of orgasm feel such distinct energy releases, they may think they have ejaculated fluid when in fact they have not.

To help attain this type of orgasm: when you feel the semen rise and you are almost at the point of no return (this is the moment you want to speed up and go faster), instead, relax all muscles and begin breathing rhythmically into the lower abdomen. Especially relax the buttocks, thighs, and lower belly. This will help you feel fulfilled rather than unsatisfied with this orgasm.

Those who are unfamiliar with this type of orgasm may try and force an ejaculation, continuing stimulation until they feel exhausted, without having the desired outcome—ejaculatory fluid. Like the Avalanche Orgasm, relaxing into the pleasurable sensations and letting go of goals and expectations is what makes the Tornado Orgasm an extraordinary experience of extended pleasure.

As with any direction on the wheel, having a long-lasting erection without ejaculating any semen is not considered a preferred type of orgasm. Some traditions emphasize methods to retain semen in order to conserve energy. However, because sexual energy is such a powerful force, retaining semen without proper training from a knowledgeable teacher, or overusing these techniques without understanding their purpose, can contribute to prostate, bladder, or kidney problems. Quodoushka encourages a balanced expression of orgasms around the wheel.

Hawk Expression

In the Sweet Medicine teachings, the hawk teaches us about choreography. Master of detail, the hawk is supremely aware of the entire dance of energy. This orgasm gives us insights into the desires of our lovers and lets us savor the exquisite variety of our sensual sensations.

Tornado Expression

In the whirlwind of feelings, touch, and passion that comes with sex there is always the silent eye within the great moving storm. Natives understood the power tornados have to clear away distractions and stir up stuck or dormant energy. The gift of the Tornado/Hawk Orgasm is to sweep away accumulated sluggishness. Men have this orgasm when they need to reduce stress. Wind orgasms leave you feeling completely calm and yet totally energized, the way you do after a howling thunderstorm. They give us the Huaqua of Humor.

WEST

Earthquake Orgasm

This orgasm comes with sweeping chills and shudders. The whole body quakes, yet there is a strong genital focus. This is the politically correct orgasm: it comes with a full erection, full ejaculation, and full orgasm. It is what we commonly think of when we think of a man's orgasm. However, if you look at this wheel, you may notice it is the only direction a man has a hard tipili and a full ejaculation of fluid.

Crow or Raven Expression

If you look at a raven or a crow with its effervescent shiny black luster, it's not hard to see why Native Americans call these birds the keepers of magic. Like them, the Crow or Raven Orgasm can be elusive, seeming to be on the verge of appearing only to manifest again in another splurge of explosive energy.

Earthquake Expression

Earthquakes are nature's way of reminding us of life's impermanence. What we think is immovable moves, and what we think is unshakeable, shakes. These orgasms restore our physical bodies and satisfy the need for sexual release. They leave us feeling so charged with raw power we forget our shortcomings and feel totally alive with pleasure. They teach us about the mysterious resilience of the human body and give us the Huaqua of Health.

EAST

Raging Forest Fire Orgasm

All I can say is that we weren't expecting this to happen. It was midwinter, but we were hotly drenched in sweat. It felt like I literally had an electric wire hooked up to my whole body, and I was red all over. I was unbelievably turned on. Even though my penis was on fire, it never got hard. It didn't stop us, though; because there was so much passion, it felt like every time we touched, more sparks would fly. I'm not sure what it was, but I know it was good.

STEPHAN, AGE FORTY-NINE

This is an East, fire orgasm. It comes with dry flashes of heat radiating from the genitals that produce sweat across the entire body. As Stephan describes, it feels like an electric current is flowing between you and your partner. There is no erection and no ejaculation, yet the body experiences a series of full orgasmic energy releases. Once again, if couples realize what is happening and do not try to induce the expected results, the Forest Fire Orgasm can take you into realms of sensation not commonly experienced.

Eagle Expression

The eagle is one of the most sacred of all the birds to indigenous people. It flies higher than any other and is thus said to carry our prayers and messages to Spirit. The Eagle Orgasm lifts lovers into soaring heights where physical limitations are transformed into pure creative energy. Men have Eagle Orgasms to access freedom and originality.

Forest Fire Expression

Fire Orgasms are always rare gifts of spirit that allow us glimpses into the unknown. They come in quick hot flashes and can expand our awareness to give us the energy we need to lift beyond insurmountable obstacles. They give us the Huaqua of Hope.

CENTER

Thunderbird or Phoenix Orgasm Expression

The Phoenix and the Thunderbird are both mythological creatures with mystical transformative powers. They rise from seeming destruction only to return stronger and more aware of their ability to manifest their desires. The Thunderbird/Phoenix Orgasm is also called Fire Breath Orgasm. They are always gifts of spirit that allow us glimpses into the unknown. They send energy throughout our entire body and help us connect to all the worlds of Grandmother Earth. They bring us into rarely felt dimensions of pleasure and give us the Huaqua of Harmony.

FEMALE ORGASMS

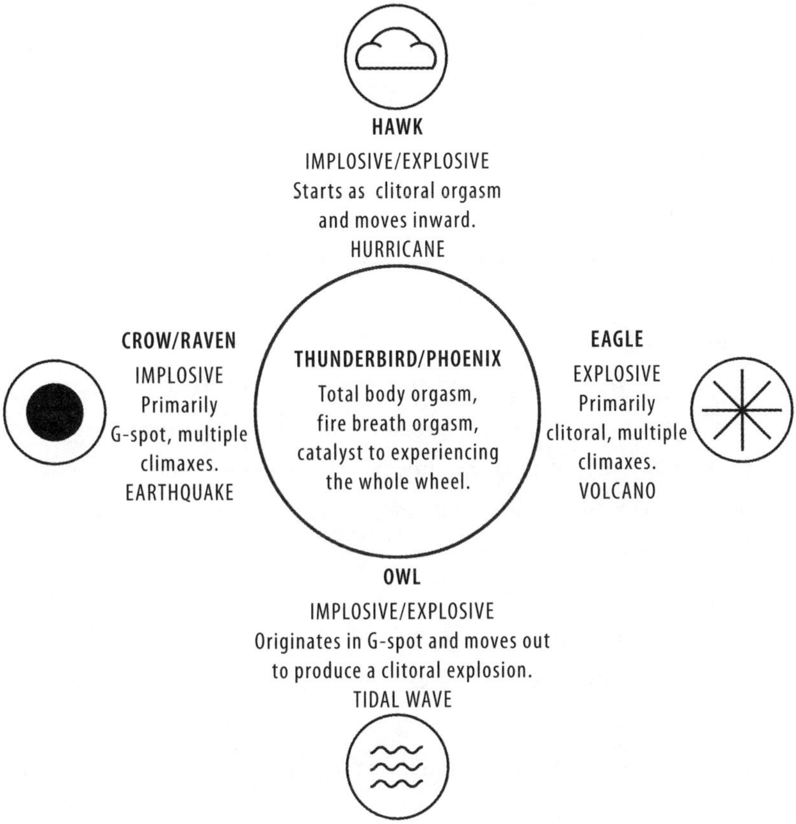

HAWK
IMPLOSIVE/EXPLOSIVE
Starts as clitoral orgasm
and moves inward.
HURRICANE

CROW/RAVEN
IMPLOSIVE
Primarily
G-spot, multiple
climaxes.
EARTHQUAKE

THUNDERBIRD/PHOENIX
Total body orgasm,
fire breath orgasm,
catalyst to experiencing
the whole wheel.

EAGLE
EXPLOSIVE
Primarily
clitoral, multiple
climaxes.
VOLCANO

OWL
IMPLOSIVE/EXPLOSIVE
Originates in G-spot and moves out
to produce a clitoral explosion.
TIDAL WAVE

Fig. 10.2. Female Orgasm Expression

SOUTH

Tidal Wave Orgasm (Implosive/Explosive)

I didn't really feel like making love when we started, but then something shifted and I really got into it. For some reason I started laughing. Pretty soon we were both laughing and still making love. It was like a faucet turned on inside, and then I started sobbing uncontrollably. I kept saying, "Please don't stop." We stayed like this, rocking, kissing, and holding each other, for a long time, I felt so close I never wanted it to end.

MARGUERITE, AGE FORTY-FOUR

This is a South, water orgasm. It originates in the Fire Trigger, G-spot area and extends more deeply within the inner cave around the cervix. It spreads out from the inside to then produce a clitoral explosion. Whether through exuberant, sometimes inexplicable laughter or through lots of tears, there is a flow of water and secretions between lovers. Any time you experience profuse emotions in recurring waves of loving intimacy and tenderness, you are having a Tidal Wave Orgasm.

Owl Expression
Owls fly silently in the night and then swoop upon their prey with absolute certainty. These orgasms begin quietly, often slipping up, surprising us with the intensity of built-up emotions that come pouring forth. The force of intimacy first draws us inward and then explodes outward in showers of emotion.

Tidal Wave Expression
Swells of feeling come in powerful surges of cresting waves. Like the undertow of an enormous wave, lovers are pulled so strongly together they merge in oceanic oneness. The gift of Tidal Wave/Owl Orgasms is to wash away self-doubt, fear, and insecurity; they make us feel beautiful to the core of our being. Feelings, love, and exquisite tenderness envelop us until we can taste

the sweetness of life. As with the male expression, the South Orgasm for women ultimately leaves us feeling filled with the Huaqua of Happiness.

NORTH

Hurricane Orgasm (Explosive/Implosive)

We started with a fantasy I had about being blindfolded during oral sex. My partner started playing with my clitoris. It got so intense I started having these wisps whip through me over and over again that kept getting stronger and stronger. I was screaming and thrashing because everything felt so incredible. Having a blindfold on was amazing because I didn't know what was coming next. We were insatiable. I wanted something deep inside me and I didn't want it to stop. Finally, I curled up in a little ball and just lay there shaking.

JUNIPER, AGE THIRTY-SEVEN

This is a North, wind orgasm. It begins in the clitoral area and comes in quick, multiple sensations that typically crest in several increasingly intense bursts. At some point, the energy starts to draw inward, usually culminating in a powerful, sometimes sudden implosion. It is often accompanied by passionate conversation, erotic talk, or arousing playfulness. Fantasy, teasing, and surprises heighten these orgasms. We sometimes have a Hurricane Orgasm when we are feeling mentally stuck, dull, or confused about something in our lives.

Hawk Expression

The rasping scream of these keen-eyed raptors conveys the intensity of the Hawk Orgasm. Frequently, the whole body tenses during rising jerks and rushes of pleasure and then plunges into an orgasmic inward pull. Sometimes, at the height of a woman's pleasure, her screams of joy are as powerful as a screeching hawk.

Hurricane Expression

Hurricanes take entire cities with them in their torrents of whirling energy. When a woman has a Hurricane Orgasm, once she is sufficiently stimulated, she takes off on her own and becomes unstoppable. It's as if the layers of teasing and seduction generate so much internal force they finally lift the body into soaring bliss.

The gift of the Hurricane/Hawk Orgasm is to liberate us from tension, constraints, and built-up stress. It awakens brilliance and clarity in our minds and leaves us feeling swept clean of worry and doubt. Sometimes, in the aftermath of a North orgasm, we end up laughing and feeling lighter, refreshed, and ready to begin new things.

WEST

Earthquake Orgasm (Implosive)

I felt like the bed was rising and falling. We were so connected I could feel him inside as if he were actually touching my heart with his penis. We would stay like this for a while, rest a few minutes, and then start all over again. I don't know how long we made love, and I lost count of how many orgasms I had. My belly was still shaking hours later.

LEELA, AGE THIRTY-ONE

This orgasm is a West, Earthquake Orgasm. It originates inside as a rolling feeling in the womb. Like the rumbling of an earthquake starting with milder sensations, it builds gradually in strength until it implodes inside with great force. These deeply satisfying orgasms induce swells of gratitude and profound intimacy. Earthquake Orgasms invigorate our bodies, and they usually come in multiple climaxes with numerous aftershocks. Aftershocks are the involuntary quakes and shakes our body makes following an orgasm. They can last several minutes up to about an hour or more after intense lovemaking.

Crow or Raven Expression

The raven and crow are the keepers of magic. They are highly sociable and tend to be ravenous eaters. Like the sometimes clever, mysterious tricksters they are, West orgasms can sneak up on you and take you by surprise. These orgasms allow us to feel the body's magical ability to restore the Huaqua of Health.

Earthquake Expression

Grandmother Earth moves her vast tectonic plates to shift and move her "body." The deep cracks that open in the ground may seem frightening to us, and Earth's shaking can bring entire buildings down in moments. Yet earthquakes allow Earth to breathe and are extremely healing for the planet.

The gift of the Earthquake/Raven Orgasm is to take us beyond superficial connections into the rich layers of intimacy and love. When we have this kind of orgasm, it signals we need energetic physical movement. We literally need to be shaken to the core. It also means that we should listen more to our body's desire for intimate touch and sexual release.

EAST

Volcano Orgasm (Explosive)

This was a totally unexpected experience for my partner and me. It started when we were just kissing one night. For some reason it felt like his lips were on fire and I couldn't stop kissing him. We were like two electric wires—all we had to do was kiss and the sparks started to fly. I felt like my whole body kept exploding like a rocket. The more we made love, the hotter it got. It felt like my pussy was on fire. We had so much energy we were drenched in sweat, and we wanted more. I completely lost count of how many times I came, and it didn't matter.

VAUDA, AGE THIRTY-TWO

This is an East, fire orgasm. It is primarily focused around the clitoris and is marked by increasingly intense, quick, and passionate bursts of multiple climaxes. The woman's expressions are expansive and vast. Once the molten heat starts to stir and rise, it feels as if she lifts upward into the stars. We often have a Volcano/Eagle Orgasm when we need connection to the positive, creative, cosmic forces of life.

Eagle Expression

Some eagles perform an elaborate mating ritual called cartwheeling, in which they lock talons high in midair, flip into a free fall for hundreds of yards, and then separate only a few yards before hitting the ground. Then they soar upward to do it again. Eagle Orgasms are equally exhilarating states of ecstasy with numerous climaxes.

Volcano Expression

Like a volcano's seemingly slow, oozing buildup of molten heat that brews and escalates for years, these orgasms are the result of mounting seduction and desire. They produce extremely passionate explosions of healing force. When a woman has a Volcano Orgasm, she reaches into the highest aspects of herself. Burning away impurities, she leaves a trail of exalted purity and tranquility to follow.

The gift of the Eagle/Volcano Orgasm is to take lovers into expansive flights of bliss where they can breathe in fresh insights, gather inspirations, and illuminate their deepest desires. They fill our spirits with the Huaqua of Hope.

CENTER

Fire Breath Orgasm (Same for Men and Women)

Please read chapter 12 for a better understanding of this orgasm. Until it is experienced, it is hard to believe that while practicing the Fire Breath the entire body can reach a full orgasmic climax without any outward genital stimulation whatsoever. The intensely pleasurable sensations that ripple and course throughout the body are activated by breath, muscle control, and mental intention. The total body orgasm that issues forth is not localized in the genitals.

The Fire Breath Orgasm is the catalyst (along with the Heart-Pleasuring Exercise) to increase the intensity and level of our orgasms. Like all the other types, the Fire Breath Orgasm is extremely healing. It helps invigorate and balance the various energy systems throughout the body. Practicing the Fire Breath enhances the restorative healing benefits for every type of orgasm on the wheel. It can also be helpful for "preorgasmic" men who experience premature ejaculation and for women who experience low levels of sexual desire. Finally, because the Fire Breath Orgasm is not subject to the ordinary limitations of the physical body, those who wish to experience multiple climaxes should learn this technique from a qualified teacher.

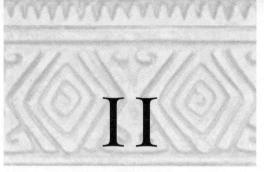

11

Increasing the
Intensity of Orgasms

*Orgasms are one of the most misunderstood expressions of
the human body. We tend to make having them far too
complicated and thus lose many of their healing benefits.*

Quodoushka answers the question, What are orgasms for? by stating first
and foremost: they are for our health. Native wisdom and common sense
remind us that our bodies need orgasms as much as we need to eat and
sleep. Being able to enjoy them is a measure of good health. When we are
sick or depressed, we not only lose our appetite for food, our desire for sex
comes to a halt too, and we avoid stimulus to conserve our energy. Having
an orgasm when we are weak seems out of the question because we think
it will drain our energy, and for the most part, when we think this way,
it does. Quodoushka turns around the belief that orgasms rob us of vital
energy and shows how the opposite can be true if we understand what
makes us gain and lose energy.

ORGASMS THAT GIVE US ENERGY

Of course, having an orgasm does not readily cure every ill, and if we are
seriously ill, we don't have energy for sex. However, if we want to stay

healthy, a regular diet of orgasmic release is one of the things that keeps us well. Recent scientific studies confirm that sexual stimulation can relieve a range of illnesses, from the common cold to the pain of arthritis. Some tests suggest the absorption of semen acts like an antidepressant. Other research shows that various mood-enhancing hormones such as endorphins, serotonins, and gonadotropins are released into the bloodstream whenever we have an orgasm. It turns out these chemicals trigger different regions of our brains and cause us to feel good. While it is becoming scientifically clear that our orgasms stimulate the production of certain chemicals, Quodoushka looks beyond the hormonal benefits in stating that orgasms give us emotional, physical, mental, spiritual, and sexual balance and harmony as well.

LOSING ENERGY WITH SEX

When we use them well, our orgasms can sustain our health and well-being. Yet it is also true we can lose energy by having low-level orgasms. Our orgasms are either a source of sweet medicine in our lives, helping us feel more joyful, connected, and hopeful about life, or they become a source of frustration. Our attitude and approach to sex has a lot to do with how healing our orgasms are, and there are ways we can actually be depleted by our sexual exchanges. If we are obsessed with sexual thoughts, try to press our demands on others, complain about not having enough, or blame someone for our dissatisfaction, the benefits of orgasms turn against us. We can also lose energy by staying stuck in unsatisfying relationships in which we cannot express what's missing. Eventually we will shut down, withdraw, and start gathering resentments. Although we may love our partner, when these kinds of disappointments accumulate, we get discouraged, turned off, and feel drained. Rather than being a vital medicine, until we find a way to have more satisfying experiences, sexual intimacy turns into a kind of poison.

Although we will not cease to exist if we do not have an orgasm for a while, gradually our lack of desire for intimate connection weakens our life-force energy. When we neglect the body's need for sexual expression, or we deny ourselves orgasms for too long, sooner or later, our health suffers. We become lethargic and age more quickly. Quodoushka views sex not only as the most important way we bond intimately with our lovers, it sees our ability to enjoy high-level orgasms as being an accurate measure of our overall health. When we are feeling low, finding a way to express ourselves sexually is an excellent way to restore our vitality.

HAVING HIGHER-LEVEL ORGASMS

When it comes to measuring the strength of an orgasm, the best way is to start considering them "all good." As Yogi Berra reportedly said, "When sex is good it's fabulous, and when it's not so good, it's still pretty good." While sharing only mild orgasmic pleasure with someone can be lovely, there is no question having a powerful orgasm is one of the greatest feelings there is. In general, when we experience high-level orgasms more consistently, our health increases, and if we mostly have low-level orgasms, it means we have some work to do in our intimate relationships.

High-level orgasms take us into expanded states of perception where our hearts open and love flows unconditionally. We gain a direct connection to the Source and feel oneness with everything. This is the magical state of creational awareness in which two life-force energies come together to generate a new energy—the Quodoushka energy—which can be used for healing or manifesting desires into physical reality. Mind you, even a fast, brief encounter can take you to the point where you cannot distinguish between where one body ends and the other begins. Sometimes our best orgasms happen when we least expect them.

Mostly, we'd like to have great orgasms and avoid the mediocre ones. We want the benefits without putting out much effort. We think, as long as we love someone or we find the right person, sex should be fantastic. The truth is, minding our physical health plays a huge role in determining the levels of our orgasms. Without sufficient exercise, a good diet, and a balanced lifestyle, the energy we gain from sex will remain low. Paradoxically, the way to enjoy consistently higher levels of orgasm is to let go of trying to get them. Trying to have an excellent orgasm is about as useful as running a marathon without training. It won't work. Orgasms increase in strength and healing power when we pay attention to the various ways we are connecting—not only sexually with our partners, but with anyone we meet. Are we distant and aloof, or are we listening and supportive? Are we stressed and tense, or are we playful and open?

Increasing the level of our orgasms is a matter of improving our entire lifestyle. Most importantly, the more present and responsive we are to our lover's needs and the more spontaneity we bring to our love life, the higher the level of orgasm we will experience.

It is actually the neutral perception of what is called the Observer Witness that increases the strength of our orgasms. This is because, as we calmly observe the energy of our lovemaking without attachment to the past or expecting a certain outcome, we begin to savor what *is* happening more than what we project or pretend is going to happen. Even though we may desire Earth-shattering ecstatic orgasms every single time, the secret to having them more often is to slow down, calm the mind, and pay close attention to the openings for intimacy.

THE TWO PHASES OF SEXUAL AROUSAL

During various stages of orgiastic arousal, there is a measure of *charge* and *discharge*. Understanding these phases will help you see how you can build, store, and properly release orgasmic energy to increase your vitality. The *charge* of an orgasm is the energy it takes to build toward climax. The *discharge* is the amount of energy released during and after climax.

The Charge

If the charge we build up in approaching an orgasm is insufficient, the energy we release will be weak. In other words, if what it takes to have an orgasm is too difficult, we will feel tired rather than energized. If we neglect sexual playfulness and spontaneity, we accumulate very little charge. The message here is to enjoy the entire approach toward sex, including the foreplay, conversation, seduction, and what Quodoushka calls Building the Prey. When the entire charge of stimulation is lighthearted and unattached, it always increases our energy. Whether we reach orgasm or not is of little importance. The "prey" we are seeking is neither the orgasm nor the energy from our partner. The real secret of building the charge is to let go of the goal and enjoy the ride no matter what it looks like. While it takes determination, Building the Prey should be spontaneous and fun. The "prey" is the dance between you and your partner, and orgasms are the gifts of your union.

The Discharge

When we have an orgasm, we discharge, or release the energy we have built up. If we do not feel much of an energy gain after having an orgasm, it is because we have built up a low charge (we were not highly stimulated), and therefore the discharge is minimal. Generally, we gain energy if the discharge is equal to or greater than the charge. Thus, without sufficient stimulation, we cannot have a high-level orgasm. Having many discharges without building a sufficient charge weakens our vitality. It is important to keep in mind that we can have different kinds of orgasmic release. Creating a balance of charge and discharge, by using the practices in this book and enjoying a variety of sexual experiences, is what ultimately leads to better health.

THE LAWS OF ENERGY MOVEMENT

Natural Energy Laws

Quodoushka measures the level of an orgasm by observing the kind of energy it produces. After having an orgasm, we experience various degrees of closeness or separation. For example, sometimes after an orgasm we actually feel somewhat distant from our partner and may want to turn away even though the sex was okay. Other times we feel a bit closer, yet still feel only mildly satisfied. After other climaxes we feel totally energized. At these higher levels of orgasm, we want to talk, touch, kiss, and caress, and at even higher levels, we merge so fully we dissolve into

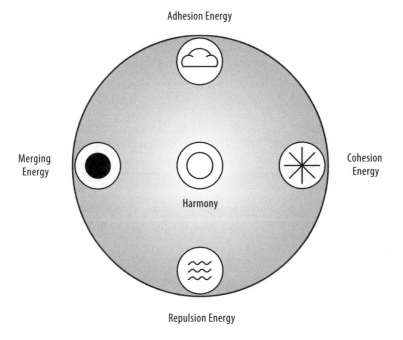

Fig. 11.1. Laws of Energy Movement

each other until we become completely inseparable. At higher levels, our lovemaking generates energy. We are so tuned in to every sensation; we can hear the thoughts of our lover, and it feels like we could make love indefinitely.

The following teaching shows us how to recognize the different laws of energy our orgasms produce. While making love, we will experience each of these laws of energy very quickly. For example, within one sexual encounter there will be brief moments of separation, closeness, or profound connection. These energies constantly move through our sexual relationships, regardless of how much we love our partner. Every orgasm can thus be measured, not for the purpose of comparing, but rather to help us reach deeper states of sexual union.

Repulsion Energy

Repulsion energy is separation. If we are experiencing a moment of repulsion, we may even have a slight feeling of irritation after making love.

This means that rather than generating closeness, our orgasm actually leaves us feeling tired or more separated than when we began. It is easy to be discouraged when we feel repulsion energy. However, if you see it as a temporary wave that sometimes happens, rather than sinking and separating more, you can change the energy by deliberately giving more affection. An example of a positive side of repulsion energy would be when we go on vacation. The separation actually makes us delighted to reunite.

Adhesion Energy

With adhesion energy, we feel temporary bonds that come and go. With a weak bond, a connection may be friendly and casual, but the minute anything happens we do not like, we are easily pulled back into our own self-focus. Adhesion energy is also the energy we use to explore attractions, create rapport, and share easygoing, lighthearted connections. With a lover, when adhesion energy is present, we are questioning whether we want to make love or not. We frequently bond through friendly gestures of affection and by sharing things we love to do. The key to taking moments of adhesion into a deeper sexual experience is to totally enjoy the things you do together.

Change Energy

Change energy is always present. Within every sexual encounter, the dynamic between partners can quickly move from repulsion, to adhesion, to cohesion, and back again to adhesion. These dynamics are called laws because they describe how energy is operating. The only predictable thing about sexual energy is that it will change. That's its beauty.

Cohesion Energy

Cohesion energy is what we like to feel after an orgasm; it's when we generate so much charge that we want to make love for hours. We surrender into euphoric dreams only to wake with the desire to do it again. We start to feel timeless, ageless, and even genderless. The boundary between our single bodies disappears; there is no separation. Our total cohesion catalyses creative ideas, laughter, dreams, joy, contentment, and hope.

THE FOUR LEVELS OF ORGASM

The constant motion of these laws of energy determines which level of orgasm we will experience.

Level-One Orgasm

The Energy Movement: Repulsion Energy

With a level one orgasm, partners feel distant and separate. Even though the man may ejaculate and the woman may climax, their lovemaking is distracted and routine. Neither has much desire to connect, but they stay in there. Both partners have to work hard and put out too much in order to have sex. When there is finally a climax, it's ho-hum. There is very little charge, a good discharge with little or no gain of energy and sometimes even a loss of energy. Partners feel sleepy and tired and do not want to continue. One or the other typically rolls over and falls asleep.

EMOTIONALLY

The woman wants to be held and cuddled. She may crave affection, but she withdraws.

The man wants to be left alone. He does not want to touch or kiss. He is aloof and remote.

MENTALLY

The woman is semi-talkative, but she is self-absorbed.

The man is distracted and also focused on his own pleasure. He is off in another world, thinking about other matters.

PHYSICALLY

The woman experiences about three to eight involuntary contractions lasting thirty seconds to two minutes. Her body is somewhat satisfied, vaguely wanting more, but she is too tired to continue.

The man has an average of three to five spurts of ejaculate, or releases of energy, lasting about twenty to thirty seconds. Afterward, he is tired and wants to sleep.

Spiritually and Sexually

The woman is somewhat relaxed and clear. She is slightly intuitive, but she is unsatisfied and closed.

The man is in a neutral state. He feels empty and is devoid of sexual responsiveness.

Chakra Level Reached (See chapter 12)

(This means the indicated chakras are opening with moving energy circulating through them.)

The woman: First through third chakras

The man: First chakra

The Shields (See chapter 12)

The woman's Little Girl, Child Substance Shield* is balanced. Her Adult Woman's Shield is partially experienced. This means that while the female partner feels comfortable and safe emotionally, she is not entirely satisfied physically. Although she may desire to connect, she is easily distracted and remains distant.

The man's Little Boy, Male Substance Shield† is balanced. This means that while the male partner feels somewhat satisfied physically, he withdraws and focuses on himself.

---

*The term "Substance Shield" (described in chapter 12) refers to an aspect of the energy network of the body that contains the emotional and energetic qualities of the male (Little Boy) or female (Little Girl).

†The differences between the chakras men and women activate: Quodoushka teaches that from the vantage point of pure energy movement, feminine energy leads masculine energy. This is a powerful message for anyone who wishes to understand how sexual energy functions. In brief, it does not mean women are more advanced; it actually means that being receptive and open (feminine energy) creates the conditions for higher states of pleasure. When feminine, receptive energy is met by sufficient active masculine energy, the marriage of the two produces something greater than either individual energy.

It also means that if a woman is insufficiently aroused, only low-level orgasms can occur.

Level-Two Orgasm

The Energy Movement: Repulsion Toward Adhesion Energy

At level two, there is more physical satisfaction and a small gain of energy. There is a balance between the charge and discharge of energy. Partners experience a mild release and feel somewhat balanced in their minds and spirits. There is the beginning of a brief heart connection and a feeling of fulfillment.

EMOTIONALLY

The woman is more giving and nurturing. She wishes to caress, hold, and kiss her lover.

The man wants to be held, touched, or cuddled. He wants to listen and be talked to.

MENTALLY

The woman is contemplative and meditative. She starts to be creative and desires to work things out.

The man is somewhat talkative, open, and responsive. He has a dreamy alertness.

PHYSICALLY

The woman experiences more intense mini- though mild aftershocks with involuntary convulsions lasting about two to four minutes. Her body is glowing, flushed, and tingling. She is extremely sensitive and hyperactive. She typically wants to get up and eat, dance, and be active. The man's body is partially satisfied, but he feels he could do it again. As the energy fluctuates between repulsion and adhesion, after resting, he may try to initiate another round. Although her body is partially satisfied, she does not have quite enough energy to continue sexual play, and thus she alternately comes close and then moves away.

The man has an average of six to eight spurts of ejaculate, or releases of energy, lasting about forty to sixty seconds. Afterward, he may want to get up and move or do something active before going to sleep.

SPIRITUALLY AND SEXUALLY

The woman is beginning to be aware of her sacred dream and feels hope about things she would like to do in her life. If she goes into her own world, at level two she will be satisfied and will not extend her orgasms further.

The man is tranquil, relaxed, and clear, but he is reluctant to allow the feminine energy to lead. Both typically separate and start thinking about other things.

CHAKRA LEVEL REACHED

The Woman: First through fifth chakras

The Man: First, second, and third chakras

THE SHIELDS (SEE CHAPTER 12)

The woman feels her Adult Woman's Shield and has a slight awareness of her Adult Spirit Man Shield. This means that she has had a fairly satisfying sexual release and begins to feel more active and creative.

The man feels his Adult Man Shield, but is still partially in his Little Boy, Child Substance Shield. This means that while he has had a good sexual release, he may be emotionally sensitive, insecure about his performance, and still slightly distant.

Level-Three Orgasm

The Energy Movement: Adhesion Toward Cohesion Energy

At level three, there is a great deal of fulfillment and connection in our emotions, minds, bodies, spirits, and sexual hungers. We feel open and extremely playful, having quickly ascending, intensely powerful charges and extended discharges with multiple climaxes. (These can be felt as tremors and waves of extended pleasure.) Both partners experience a distinct energy gain. As our male and female energies finally align, we let go of our bodies' limitations while reaching for more. We become expressive and highly creative. Healing and spontaneous insights begin at this level. If we try something sexually new by using any of the Lovers'

Masks (see chapter 13), the intimacy and intensity of orgasms will lift even higher.

Emotionally

Both partners want to stroke, hold each other, and cuddle. There is happiness and camaraderie. In the joy of being together we feel desired, cherished, and beautiful. We share a great deal of laughter and curiosity and want to explore more together.

Mentally

For both, images of past lives may appear. We may see face changes and slip in and out of the dream together. Conversation becomes highly intimate and affirming. Each has a desire to help manifest the other's aspirations.

Physically

The body is alive and humming. Both partners are vibrating and wish to make love again.

> The woman has many strong, extended aftershocks with extremely powerful discharges. She may have multiple types of orgasms.

> The man has a powerful release, can recover his energy, and in some cases may have several types of orgasms, with or without ejaculate.

Spiritually and Sexually

The sexual energy generated is so moving it kindles feelings of harmony and resonance with all the worlds: the sun, moon, stars, plants, animals, minerals, ancestors, and humans. This is where we expand beyond our potential awareness and gain insights into how we can contribute our gifts to the collective dream. Sometimes we feel a driving passion. We become lusty and insatiable, yet we are deeply fulfilled. We both have extended waves of orgasmic pleasure, with many aftershocks. Neither of us is sure which feels better: our own pleasure or our partner's.

Ideally, to balance all five aspects, emotionally, mentally, physically, spiritually, and sexually, this (or at least a level 2.5) is the level of orgasm we should seek to enjoy. Note: At times lovers will experience the same level of orgasm, while at other times there will be a slight difference. Mostly, we are in close range with our partner's level of orgasm. It is important to keep in mind that we can always shift into higher gear the moment we reach for a Light Arrow and give with tenderness. It is always possible to raise the level of orgasm by returning to a balanced use of our energy.

CHAKRA LEVEL REACHED

The Woman: First through seventh chakras

The Man: First through fifth chakras

THE SHIELDS (SEE CHAPTER 12)

The woman experiences the Adult Spirit Man Shield. This is where a woman feels almost as if she has a penis and vice versa. A woman sexually awakens her creative, active conceptive energy.

The man experiences the Adult Woman Spirit Shield. This is where the man becomes open, relaxed, and totally receptive. With very high states of orgasm, he can feel as if he has a vagina. The more each partner dips into the opposite gender, the more attraction they have for each other. This generates feelings of driving, insatiable passion.

Level-Four Orgasm

The Energy Movement: Cohesion Energy

At level four we feel completely fulfilled and are in the "zone." Lovers merge in all five aspects and can go on, extending their connection through and beyond intercourse. The duration of discharges, including tingling, shaking, and the desire to connect, are greatly extended. The charge fuels the discharge and the discharge fuels the charge, creating an infinite loop of magical cosmic force. All time and sense of limitation disappear, and any type of orgasm can happen. Our movements become tranquil and our stillness vibrates until we begin over and over again. Even through dreaming, there are no longer two separate bodies. Only the pure sensation of being lovingly connected to everything exists.

EMOTIONALLY

We feel expanded understanding and compassion with all creation. Our hearts, bodies, and minds unite in openness and loving light. The five Huaquas of Health, Hope, Happiness, Harmony, and Humor are awakening in us, and we are filled with the desire to give.

MENTALLY

At this level, our orgasms induce our natural gifts to come forth. We gain access to the memory of talents, skills, and abilities from other lifetimes and become exceptionally aware of the power of our thoughts. We experience profound intuitions about what our lover needs and instinctively know precisely what to do and say. Past and future merge completely into the present.

PHYSICALLY

At this level aging slows or stops entirely. Healing and physical transformations occur spontaneously. It becomes clear that our bodies are in our minds. Illumination and light extend everywhere, and other qualities of time, space, and dimensional realities appear.

SPIRITUALLY AND SEXUALLY

During a fourth-level orgasm, we realize our true feminine and masculine wisdom. With an excruciatingly beautiful sense of gratitude, as our hearts and bodies open, we are given the energy to walk the path of our destiny. We know how we can contribute to the planetary, universal, and cosmic dream. We birth each other's potential and share the profuse love of the God and Goddess together as one.

CHAKRA LEVEL REACHED

The Woman: First through tenth chakras

The Man: First through eighth chakras; may follow the woman into the ninth and tenth

THE SHIELDS (SEE CHAPTER 12)

The woman experiences her opposite gender Little Boy, Spirit Shield.

She may move into the Goddess as she births the God.

The man experiences his opposite gender Little Girl, Spirit Shield.

SUMMARY

Experiencing more intense orgasms, where we dissolve into the pure states of ecstatic pleasure, begins with how we view the purpose of our orgasms. If we capitulate to whatever makes them so difficult to enjoy, our sexual feelings will wane and weaken. If we forget how our orgasms sustain our emotional, mental, physical, spiritual, and sexual well-being, chances are sex will fall to the very bottom of our list of things to do. The practice of Quodoushka is to remember that when we get lazy about sex and we cannot muster the energy to initiate intimate connections, we lose life force energy.

Our orgasms and the states of hypersensitivity they induce, are not only essential for our health and longevity, they take us into the gateways of awareness where we can be replenished by the light of creation. Whenever we say yes to closeness, yes to tenderness, and finally, yes to our body's desire to experience the highest states of pleasure possible, we gain energy. Saying yes to the opportunities that appear is the first step toward enjoying the remarkable healing energy of high-level orgasms.

12

SEXUAL HEALING PRACTICES

GETTING TO KNOW THE SUBTLE ENERGIES OF SEX

One of the major contributions of Quodoushka involves showing us how we can utilize the intricate network of energy that comprises and surrounds us to enhance the quality of our lovemaking. Although we may not be aware of these networks, there is undeniably something more going on than mere physical contact between two people. At the very least, we know our unseen thoughts and emotions can either raise or ruin our chances to have a beautiful encounter. But there are many other "invisible" fields of energy that come into play during sex. Well before we had brain scans and MRIs to visualize detailed internal structures of rotating magnetic fields, shamans not only developed the ability to see these types of phenomena, they learned how to guide the invisible with their intent. In simple terms, if we focus only on the physical aspects of sex, we will continue having lower-level orgasms. Once we become aware of these subtle energetic frequencies, our experience of sex can become more sensitive, and thus more fulfilling.

Most current medical models do not recognize any lights or auras around the physical body, but even as our culture gradually accepts acupuncture as an effective method to relieve pain, we have yet to build technology to show the existence of the energy channels that explain how it works. Western science describes phenomena by what it can isolate, measure, and technically magnify into perception. Since the sexual functions of desire and arousal are not easily imaged, the energy systems shamanic cultures learned to direct are likely to remain largely unexplored by mainstream science for some time.

Nevertheless, for thousands of years, naguals and sages in various ancient cultures have known that sexual energy could heal imbalances and extend life. While they may not have had technology to produce pictures of sexual arousal, their knowledge of its importance led them to develop ways to harness its power. For example, in some cultures a man returning from the sickness of a tribal war would be welcomed home with ritual lovemaking so that he could heal from grief and remorse. It was understood that the energy produced through sexual union could restore harmony in the body and heal the wounds of his spirit.

SEXUAL ENERGY HEALING

In our culture, where the common purposes of sex are to attract a mate, maintain partnerships, have children, or have a great time, using sexual energy for healing is still somewhat of a foreign concept. Sex in the West is not often viewed as a means to generate a substantial healing force, and thus the power of sexual intimacy to heal physical, emotional, or psychological imbalances is not well understood. Furthermore, whenever sexual energy is used in selfish or manipulative ways, the restorative qualities of sex cannot be accessed. The key to understanding how to utilize sexual energy for healing is to start to see, sense, and feel the various aspects of our energy light network that comprise and surround our physical bodies.

At the first levels of awareness, we are so busy dealing with all the emotional issues that come with having or not having sex, we seldom notice anything beyond our desire for gratification. As we evolve into potential awareness, even if we cannot see our energetic bodies yet, we begin to sense that there are other dimensions to sexual intimacy. Expanding our perception to include the energetic aspects of our being allows us to feel the needs and desires of our partners. We not only have more intense sexual feelings and higher-level orgasms, as the vibrancy of our energy bodies increase, sex naturally becomes more healing.

THE HUMAN FLOWERING TREE OF LIFE

Ultimately, every cell in our being has one purpose: to realize its full potential and return to the original nature of pure Spirit. Like a tree whose roots sink into the So Below of Earth, and whose branches reach into the As Above of the sky, our evolution into formlessness and our entire journey to realize who we truly are is symbolized by the growing branches, trunk, roots, and blossoms of a flowering tree. The components of the complete spectrum of our energy bodies are called Human Flowering Trees. Here we will consider only a few aspects. The Human Flowering Tree actually contains Five Senses, Ten Eyes, Five Ears, Five Evolutionary States of Consciousness, Four Attentions, Five Shields, Seven Dancers, an Octagonal Mirror, Three Assemblage Points, and various Filament Fibers, to name a few. Each component plays a unique role in the movement of our soul's evolution toward enlightenment.

If we could actually *see* ourselves as energy, we would perceive what the Twisted Hairs call a Luminous Egg Cocoon, because the pulsating lights surrounding our physical bodies resemble a cocoon of light in the shape of an egg. Inside this human cocoon of luminosity is a microcosm of the entire planetary system filled with an amazing array of colored spheres, fibers, and filaments of swirling energy otherwise known as the chakras. The physical body, which is made of denser, more slowly moving light, rests in the center like the yolk of the egg.

THE TEN CHAKRAS

Knowledge accumulated through direct observations made by indigenous healers of Asia, India, and Mesoamerica describes vortexes or funnels that circulate the course of energy throughout the physical body. Taoists refer to these areas as cavities where energy gathers and either radiates like beaming headlights or stays clogged inside kinked-up hoses. Quodoushka refers to them as *chula,* which, like the Sanskrit word *chakra,* means a turning wheel.

For that's what chakras are—invisible to most, they are wheels of energy light that whirl like rotor blades when we're healthy, and sputter and finally stop when we die. Quodoushka explains a system of ten major

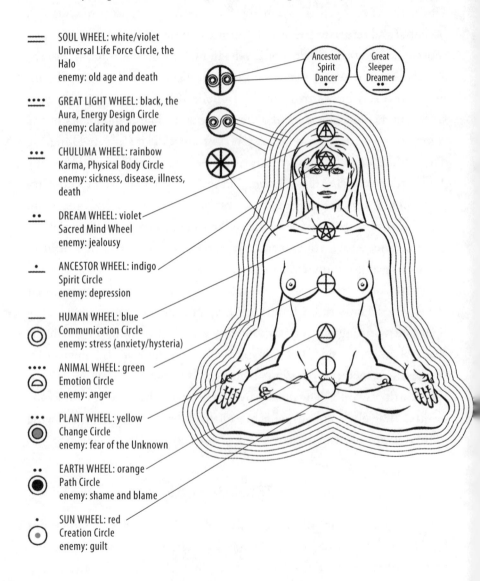

SOUL WHEEL: white/violet
Universal Life Force Circle, the Halo
enemy: old age and death

GREAT LIGHT WHEEL: black, the Aura, Energy Design Circle
enemy: clarity and power

CHULUMA WHEEL: rainbow
Karma, Physical Body Circle
enemy: sickness, disease, illness, death

DREAM WHEEL: violet
Sacred Mind Wheel
enemy: jealousy

ANCESTOR WHEEL: indigo
Spirit Circle
enemy: depression

HUMAN WHEEL: blue
Communication Circle
enemy: stress (anxiety/hysteria)

ANIMAL WHEEL: green
Emotion Circle
enemy: anger

PLANT WHEEL: yellow
Change Circle
enemy: fear of the Unknown

EARTH WHEEL: orange
Path Circle
enemy: shame and blame

SUN WHEEL: red
Creation Circle
enemy: guilt

Ancestor Spirit Dancer

Great Sleeper Dreamer

Fig. 12.1. The Ten Chakras

wheels pulsating within our Luminous Egg Cocoon. Seven are located along the central column of the body. The eighth is the physical body itself, the ninth is the aura, and the tenth is the halo of energy that forms rings of light above the head. Each corresponds to a color, influences organs, is guided by a certain planet, and has a specific purpose relating to the body's overall functioning.

Why Would You Want to Know How Your Chakras Are Doing?

The truth is, you'll live just fine even if you've never heard of a chakra. However, when you find out that feeling insecure, fearful, anxious, uncreative, or unsexy has a lot to do with sluggish chakras, the subject gets more interesting. It gets even more interesting when you learn that women's chakras turn one way and men's another. It's also one of the hidden reasons why it feels incredibly nice to have our whole body next to someone we like. It's not just our skin that touches—we also have these spinning spheres of light that act like the magnetic fields of batteries vibrating between us in opposite directions. When we are highly aroused, the spin of our chakras quickens. These energy spins can be extremely stimulating; we feel them as attractions. The same chakra energies move between same-sex partners. When two women or two men are together sexually, they are attracted to the similar rotations of energy rather than the differences.

Magnetic Attracting Thought-Space

When we see past physical appearances and begin to sense the various aspects of our luminosities, we will come to see that we are actually made of what is called a Magnetic Attracting Thought-Space comprised of electromagnetic and psychic-kinetic energy fields. Being a thought-space that is magnetically drawn to fields of bundled energy explains how we cluster together with kindred spirits. Along with our chakras, viewing ourselves as a Magnetic Attracting Thought-Space explains why we are irresistibly attracted to some people and uninterested in others. We gravitate toward those who emit robust electromagnetic, psychic-kinetic energy, and we create lasting friendships with people who resonate at similar energetic frequencies.

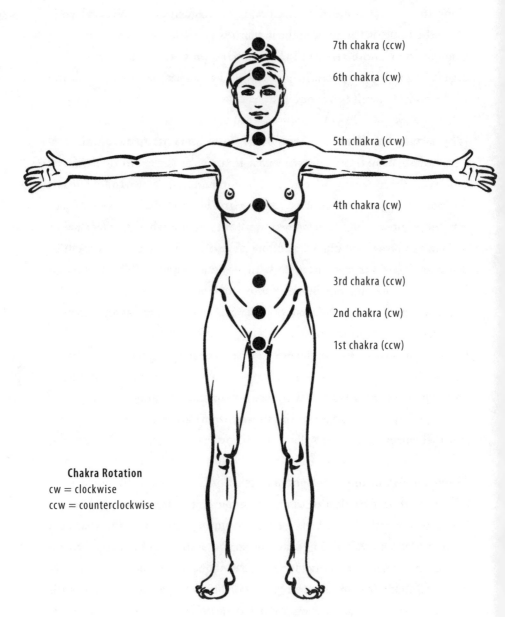

Fig. 12.2. Female Chakra Rotations

Because your body is within your mind, as you increase your magnetic thought-space (by doing things you love), your chakras surge with gusto, and you literally become more magnetic. People want to get to know you because you are flexible, vibrant, charismatic, and attractive. When chakras are listless and slow, accidents happen more frequently, you are easily exhausted, and everything seems more difficult. Because the network of interconnected energy is completely responsive, everything we do or think about doing affects the vitality of our chakras. Denying ourselves intimate sexual expression is the major way we invite the "enemies" of the chakras to interfere with the natural movement of energy throughout our bodies.

The Ten Enemies That Block Our Chakras

Life begins and ends at the first chakra located at our genitals. It's where our sexual, creative energy collects. It is called the Sun Wheel because when it's open and spinning with strength, the energy from the first chakra attracts intimacy and love. What blocks the course of our sexual, creative sun energy is the enemy of guilt. Every time we feel guilty about our natural sexual urges, and we repress, misuse, or deny our sexual feelings, we block energy from flowing through the first chakra to the rest of our body. Since they are all connected, shutting down the first chakra obstructs the circulation of the entire system.

Here is an interesting way to feel the energy of the first chakra. For a woman, the first chakra (about a four-inch "wheel" located above the clitoris and vaginal opening) normally spins counterclockwise. When she is aroused, the energy starts to spin clockwise; when she reaches a plateau, it returns to a counterclockwise rotation. Take a breath of energy inward and it's cool, blow outward to heat your hands, and the breath is hot. Counterclockwise movement produces cooling energy; clockwise, or "sun-wise," energy produces heat. Check the temperature of a woman around her first chakra after an orgasm; she becomes very cool. The opposite is true for men. At the first stages of arousal, their first chakra (underneath the base of the shaft and around the tip of the penis) becomes hot. When they ejaculate, it becomes cool, and afterward men are once again warm

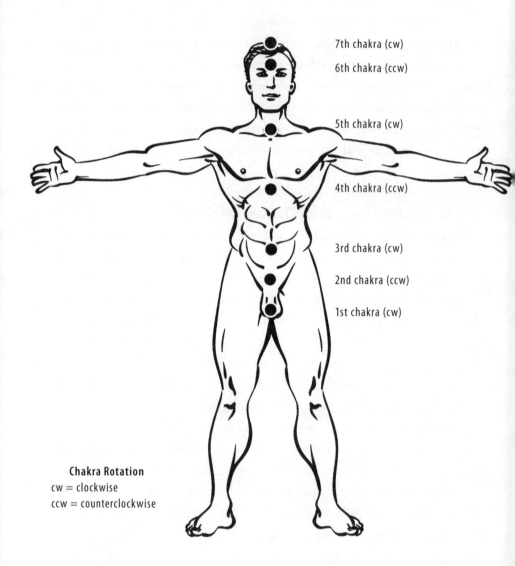

7th chakra (cw)

6th chakra (ccw)

5th chakra (cw)

4th chakra (ccw)

3rd chakra (cw)

2nd chakra (ccw)

1st chakra (cw)

Chakra Rotation
cw = clockwise
ccw = counterclockwise

Fig. 12.3. Male Chakra Rotations

at the first chakra. This means the man's energy after lovemaking returns to its natural clockwise rotation.

Look at the table on pages 224–25 to see the location, direction of rotation, correlations, and enemies of each chakra. Notice that the enemies blocking the flow of our natural energy are guilt, blame, shame, fear, stress, depression, jealousy, sickness, disease, illness, possessiveness, old age, and death. When we are enjoying sexual play, any of these enemies can enter our minds to impede the proper flow of energy through our chakras and will thus limit our charge and discharge of orgasmic energy. Although we do not experience the enemies of the chakras in any prescribed order, they originate and collect in the first chakra located around our genitals. Also notice the column labeled "Key." These are the energies that are liberated when this chakra is spinning vibrantly. Thus the key to our creativity is to increase the strength of the first chakra.

How the Enemies Invade
Our Luminous Egg Cocoon

Sustained depression slows down the sixth chakra (between the eyebrows), hindering our ability to sense or accept affection. Stress, which can be expressed as either anxiety or hysteria, constricts the fifth chakra (throat) and causes us to withdraw communication or lash out in criticism. Anger collects at the fourth chakra, around the heart, where it destroys the desire to be intimate. If we have fear at the third chakra around the navel, it is impossible to relax and feel pleasure. Shame and blame are the enemies that affect our will in the second chakra about two inches below the navel. Here, together with guilt at the first chakra, we start to feel unworthy and cannot act decisively. We are unsure about opening sexually, and if the fifth chakra (throat) stays closed, we cannot say what we dislike or ask for what we want.

All these enemies compound to diminish the potency of the seventh and tenth chakras around the top of the head, and as the first chakra grows weaker, sickness, disease and illness can enter the eighth chakra, the physical body. At this point, if we continue to suppress the need for sexual intimacy, we will strive for power, cling to attachments, and become possessive. When these enemies are left unchallenged, all the chakras rotate with less vitality, and if we remain stubborn and refuse to find a new attitude and approach we eventually succumb to feeling powerless in old age. The fear of dying becomes our greatest enemy, and it is thus impossible to face death with dignity.

These are the reasons why self-reflection ceremonies are so important to liberate our sexual energy. As we face the enemies and begin to use our lovemaking to restore the vitality of our chakras, we are literally clearing the way to allow more intimate expressions of passion to move energy through our bodies. Enjoying sex that is free from guilt, blame, or shame is one of the best ways to brighten our luminosity and keep our chakras humming.

CHAKRA, LOCATION, ENEMY, KEY

First Chakra

Location: Women: A circle 3–4 inches in diameter above the body, around the clitoris and vaginal opening

Men: Around the tip and at the base/underside of the penis

Enemy: Guilt

Key: Creativity

Second Chakra

Location: At the pubic mound, about 3–4 inches below the navel

Enemy: Shame and Blame

Key: Will and Decisiveness

Third Chakra

Location: Around the navel

Enemy: Fear (of the unknown)

Key: How we relate to change

Fourth Chakra

Location: Around the heart/sternum

Enemy: Anger (inability to cope with the unknown)

Key: Emotional balance and control

Fifth Chakra

Location: Around the throat

Enemy: Stress (cannot communicate about the inability to cope with fears)

Two expressions: Anxiety (inward, implosive), Hysteria (outward, explosive)

Key: Communication

Sixth Chakra

Location: Between the eyebrows

Enemy: Depression (unable to cope with the unknown or communicate fear or anger, we turn inward and close the Spirit Eye; a cry for valid introspection/intuition)

Key: Opening ourselves to Spirit

Seventh Chakra

Location: Top of the head

Enemy: Jealousy (inhibits our ability to dream self as a free autonomous individual)

Key: Opening our Sacred Mind

Eighth Chakra

Location: The entire body

Enemy: Sickness, Disease, Illness, Death, Possessiveness (includes envy and greed)

Key: Mastery of the physical body, health

Ninth Chakra

Location: The aura rings around the body, the Shields and the "Dancers" of our immortal soul within this incarnation (see Heart Eye in the next section)

Enemy: Clarity and Power (arrogance and self-importance)

Key: Proper design and choreography of energy within chaos

Tenth Chakra

Location: Halo rings of the aura above the head

Enemy: Old Age and Death (resistance, repression, and fear of aging and death)

Key: All things are possible

THE TEN EYES

We normally think of having two eyes and two ears to see and hear the world, but in our energetic body, we have many ways to perceive information. For example, we imagine images in the future through the third Psychic Eye, and we see images during dreams through the fifth Shadow Dream Eye. We also have "eyes" in our hands that can sense and feel. The left eye in the middle of the palm sees the essence or spirit of something; the right Dream Eye can see the potential of things. We use these energetic eyes all the time, for instance during the Pledge of Allegiance. When we place the right hand (Dream Eye) over the heart (Heart Eye), we connect the truth of our heart with the potential of our nation. The same eyes are used when we testify in a court of law, placing the left hand (Spirit Eye) on a Bible and raising the right. In this case, our Spirit Eye goes inward to see the essence, and using the Dream Eye, we vow to speak honestly.

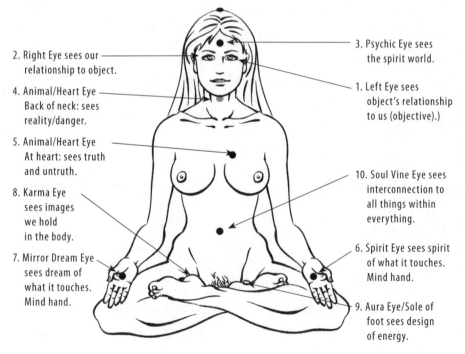

2. Right Eye sees our relationship to object.

4. Animal/Heart Eye Back of neck: sees reality/danger.

5. Animal/Heart Eye At heart: sees truth and untruth.

8. Karma Eye sees images we hold in the body.

7. Mirror Dream Eye sees dream of what it touches. Mind hand.

3. Psychic Eye sees the spirit world.

1. Left Eye sees object's relationship to us (objective).)

10. Soul Vine Eye sees interconnection to all things within everything.

6. Spirit Eye sees spirit of what it touches. Mind hand.

9. Aura Eye/Sole of foot sees design of energy.

Fig. 12.4. The Ten Eyes

The fourth eye has two functions and locations. One is at the heart, and the other is the Animal Eye located at the back of the head. This eye is open when the hairs rise on the back of your neck, because it perceives reality danger and activates instincts. We have eyes in the soles of our feet as well. Through the eighth Karma Eye of the left foot, with which drill sergeants ask soldiers to step first to march, we can perceive physical patterns. The ninth Mirror Dream Eye in the center of the sole of the right foot shows the design of energy, and it tells us when to step into the unknown. Thus in war, soldiers are asked to steady themselves with their training and skills (pattern or Karma Eye) in order to step into unknown territory (Mirror Dream Eye).

Our first and second physical eyes are the ones we know best. The left sees an object's relationship to us; the right shows our relationship to an object. The left eye perceives objectively by taking in factual information, whereas the right eye sees subjectively and gives us information about how we feel about what we see. When you are making love, if you want to connect with your feelings more, look through your right eye. To take in the fullness of your lover, gaze with both.

THE FIVE EARS

The same is true with the ears. If you wish to hear the objective facts of a situation, listen more with your left ear. If you want to hear how you feel about someone, listen with your right. The third or Middle Ear, located in the middle of our brain along with the fifth Shadow Dream Eye, not only allows us to hear voices in our dreams, it hears our inner dialogue. Our energetic eyes and ears allow us to have conversations between our Lower and Higher Selves, and they enable the various aspects within our luminosities (energy networks of moving light within and surrounding the physical body) to communicate with each other much in the same way messages travel between organs, muscles, nerves, and hormones.

The story of Ben Underwood,[1] who was said to "see" with his ears is an example of how it is possible to transcend the ordinary functions of

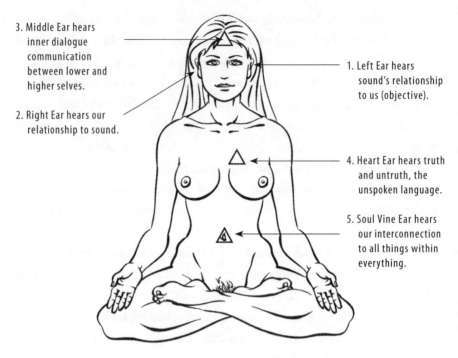

3. Middle Ear hears inner dialogue communication between lower and higher selves.

2. Right Ear hears our relationship to sound.

1. Left Ear hears sound's relationship to us (objective).

4. Heart Ear hears truth and untruth, the unspoken language.

5. Soul Vine Ear hears our interconnection to all things within everything.

Fig. 12.5. The Five Ears

our senses. Ben had his eyes removed when he was three years old because he was diagnosed with cancer. Using a process called echolocation, he learned to play basketball, surf, and skateboard through the streets by making a steady stream of sounds with his tongue, then listening for the echoes as they bounced off the surfaces around him.

On a website devoted to her son, his mother recalled that when he heard someone call somebody ugly or heard any negative comment, Ben would say, "That's what's wrong with sighted people, you all look at one another and judge what you look like." She says, "He could not judge from looks, only from spirit."[2] His mother is describing what the fourth Heart Ear does: it listens to the unspoken language of truth and untruth. In many cases, when normal sensory functions are suspended, other abilities get stronger. In Ben's case, the opening of his Heart Ear and energetic eyes enriched his extraordinary sensitivity until his recent death.

We are all capable of what the Nagual Elders call "seeing thunder and hearing lightning." In heightened states of awareness, during high-level orgasms and profound states of meditation, we transcend the limitations of our sensory perceptions. Our energetic bodies bypass what our eyes and ears normally pay attention to. When we are making love, we can open our inner ears to listen beyond careless words or negative thoughts to hear what is really longed for. We can open all our eyes to see layers of beauty with greater wisdom.

THE SOUL VINE

Located in the region around the navel are the fifth Soul Vine Ear and the tenth Soul Vine Eye. We commonly refer to these when we say, "I had a feeling in my gut something was not right." The Soul Vine Ear hears the voice of creation. The Soul Vine Eye is also called the All-Seeing Eye of the Unknown. This region is the great central hub of our being. It's the place where we receive our first nourishment and perceive our interconnection with all forms of all things. The Soul Vine Eye is actually located at the center of two energetic Fiber Filaments that extend like luminous umbilical cords from either side of the navel. They work together in absolute harmony. The left Fiber Filament is receptive/creative and sees and feels the beauty within the light; the right Fiber Filament is active/conceptive and can see the light within the darkness.

FIBER FILAMENTS

The details of Ben Underwood's life suggest something else may have been responsible for his remarkable abilities. He is recorded as the only blind person known to have developed sonar echo skills similar to dolphins. His physical hearing tested normal. Could it be he "saw with his ears" because something else was actually giving him the exact information he needed to navigate so well? Quodoushka would attribute this ability to his Fiber Filaments, which can sense and feel subtle energies that the physical senses do not register.

More than any aspect of our luminosity, the Fiber Filaments allow us to dramatically extend what we can feel within our sexual encounters. Even if you have never heard of Fibers, you have used them to gain awareness of things beyond your ordinary senses. Have you ever known someone was going to call just before the phone rang, or had a thought of someone before they died? Imagine if you could energetically feel inside your lover to peer through internal blockages to the point where you could shift stuck energy as if it were as easy as opening a closed door. With practice, that's precisely what the awareness of your Fiber Filaments gives you.

What's important to remember is that energy follows our thoughts. We can actually learn with our Fiber Filaments to connect with a lover across an ocean or to close the gap of intimacy while we are entwined in each other's arms. Unlike our physical bodies, Fiber Filaments quickly follow our unspoken intentions to connect in ways we seldom realize. At first, as with anything unseen, there's always a degree of doubt or skepticism about whether they exist at all. Nevertheless, rather than seeking dramatic results using your Fiber Filaments, it is possible to gradually gain an awareness of their presence.

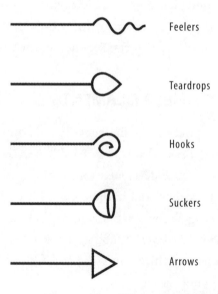

Fig. 12.6. Types of Fiber Filaments

ENERGETIC HOOKS, TEARDROPS (PROBES), SUCKERS, ARROWS, AND FEELERS (TICKLERS)

To describe them briefly, at the ends of the two major energetic Fiber Cords extending from the navel, there are twelve small variously shaped Filaments. Their shape changes according to our mind's intent. They can turn into tiny Hooks, Probes, Suckers, Arrows, or S-Shaped Feelers. These twelve energetic Filaments on each side are used to gather information in specific ways. Hooks and Suckers create attachments and dependencies, Probes touch to gather information, and Arrows can either negatively shoot anger or can be arranged internally to acquire awareness and understanding. The S-Shaped Feelers are the ones we use most during sexual play, for whether we are aware of them of not, we extend Feeler Fiber Filaments in order to connect more intimately with a lover.

Ultimately, if we are to transcend the purely physical aspects of sex and experience high-level orgasms, we also have to develop more specific ways to direct our sexual energy. The movement of our Fiber Cords and the shape of our Filaments are directed by our mind's intent and will. Thus, when we are caring and sensitive in our lovemaking, filaments automatically form into the shape of Teardrops to probe for information. When you wish to delve into intimate territory and feel much closer, they become S-Shaped. Moving and shaping the Fiber Filaments with your intention can dramatically enhance any sexual experience. You will not only become a more delicately perceptive lover, with practice, your sexual sensations increase tenfold.

In a simple experiment, try imagining two luminous cords extending from your navel. Move them in your mind up the middle of your torso and bring them over your heart. Then extend the Fiber Filaments out over the surface of your arms and into your hands. When the twelve Filaments are in your hands, imagine spreading them out in the shape of a small fan across your palms and fingers. Soon, your imagination will become reality and you will start to feel subtle currents of energy coursing through your fingertips. You can also imagine the Fiber Filaments moving downward from the navel. When they reach your genitals, spread them across your tupuli or wrap them around your tipili for greater sensuous pleasure.

THE TEACHINGS OF THE FIVE SHIELDS

There is more inside our energy bodies than you can imagine. The following diagram describes the five energetic shields contained within our Luminous Egg Cocoon. A shield is a sphere of light that filters incoming information. The Luminous Egg Cocoon contains five spheres of light that are psychic-kinetic and electromagnetic force fields of energy. These five shields keep the physical body present in third-dimensional reality. Each shield contains an identity that is an actual part of our personality which defines an aspect of who we are.

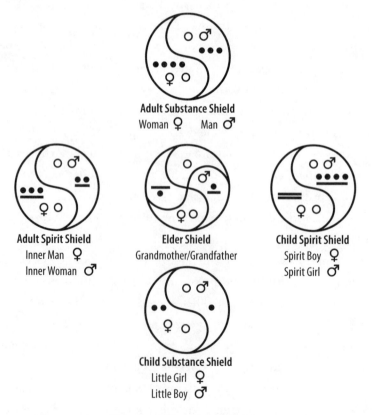

Fig. 12.7. Our Five Shields

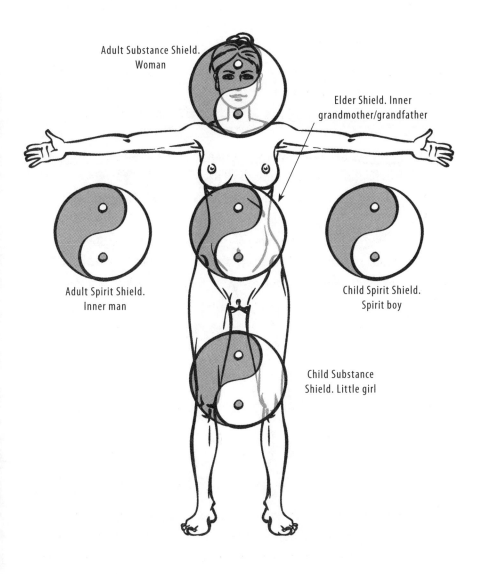

Fig. 12.8. The Five Female Shields

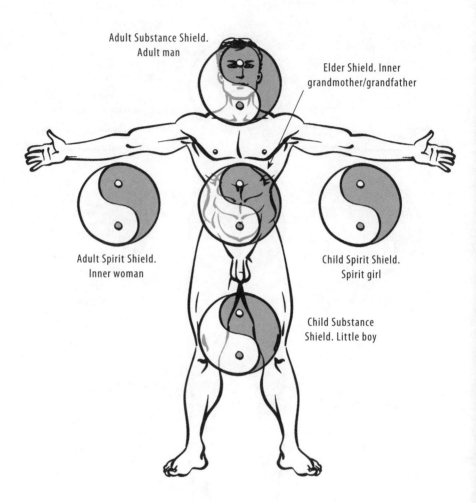

Adult Substance Shield.
Adult man

Elder Shield. Inner
grandmother/grandfather

Adult Spirit Shield.
Inner woman

Child Spirit Shield.
Spirit girl

Child Substance
Shield. Little boy

Fig. 12.9. The Five Male Shields

How the Shields Work

The five shields rotate in orbits around the body like planets. They resemble balls of light about one to three feet in diameter. Each has a male side and a female side. The large white area of the yin-yang symbol is the male side (active), and the black dot within it is the female (conceptive) within the male. The opposite is shown for the female shields.

Depending on what is happening, a different shield comes to the forefront of our luminosity, shifting the others behind and to the sides like balls on a billiard table. Whichever sphere moves to the front of the body acts like a shield that causes us to perceive incoming information in certain ways. Each shield absorbs information differently and has a unique function. While you may have never actually seen your shields, you most certainly have felt their effects. For example, although you might be in your forties, if someone extremely attractive comes near, you may suddenly feel yourself revert to childlike mannerisms. What's happening? Your Child Substance Shield has spun into the forefront of your luminosity. It is as if you now see the world through the rose-colored glasses of a little boy or a little girl. Your language and even your body movements change. Suddenly, the Child Substance Shield of your Little Boy or Little Girl is running the show, filtering your perceptions and causing you to act in certain ways. If you have ever felt "spun out," you will have felt the spinning of your shields.

There are several things to observe in these Shield Portraits. The yin-yang symbols reflect that energetically, each of our shields comprises both male and female energy. This explains how some women can appear more masculine, or men can be more feminine. They are expressing more of the male or female sides of their shields.

While the diagram shows perfect circles, in reality, the shields make the Luminous Egg Cocoon much more lopsided. If we were in perfect health and utilizing the full potential of human energy in total masculine-feminine balance, then our Shield Portrait would look like the drawing. For most, however, because it gets much more attention, the Child Substance Shield is huge, while the Child Spirit Shield is about the size of an orange. Further, because our masculine and feminine energies are imbalanced, the yin-yang portions are also greatly skewed. The key to our evolution is male-female balance. The balancing of our shields happens as a result of maintaining proper emotional, mental, physical, and spiritual choreography while learning to be both receptive and creative in our sexuality.

The Substance Shields

THE CHILD SUBSTANCE SHIELD: THE LITTLE BOY AND LITTLE GIRL

The Child Substance Shield contains memories of everything that has ever happened to us from birth through puberty. Up until the time of puberty, this shield is in the front of our luminosity, miming, mimicking, absorbing, learning, and recording everything it possibly can. It is collecting and storing both empowering "light" and wounding "dark" information. Whenever we feel hurt or rejected sexually, or get moody and clingy, we are operating from the perspective of the Child Substance Shield. The problem with being in our South Little Girl or Little Boy shields when we are faced with a sexual situation is that we cannot interact as mature adults.

THE ADULT SUBSTANCE SHIELD: THE ADULT WOMAN AND MAN

During puberty, as boys and girls we not only go through pronounced behavioral and biological changes, we also have a dramatic shift in our energetic bodies. The South Child Substance Shield moves from its front-row seat to the back, and the North Adult Substance Shield rotates over the head to the front. The Adult Substance Shield looks toward the future. Once this movement of the shields occurs within the luminosity, the proper place for childish reactions is behind us, along with the defenses we learned to protect ourselves with as kids. As we shall see later, however, when intense sexual issues confront us, the Child Substance Shield comes out front, and we cannot get past our childish ways.

The Adult Substance Shield could be called the adult "worrier." Its job is to learn what it needs to make it in the world. Through the filters of the Adult Substance Shield, as adult men and women, we choose what

kind of career, family, friends, and interests, as well as the kind of partner, we would like to have. The maturation of our Adult Woman and
Man Shield, however, is severely hindered by all the unresolved issues
contained in our Child Substance Shield. The wounds we suffered as little boys and girls produce an angry, revengeful, and manipulative Adult
Substance Shield. Regardless of our age, sexual conflicts are a result of
the struggle between our needy, wounded, and abandoned Little Boy/
Girl Shields and our angry, revengeful, and manipulative Adult Man/
Woman Shields. Whenever we are anxious about what's going to happen, lash out in resentment or jealousy, or try to control our partner,
we are operating from the dark side of our Adult Substance Shield. All
the dramas and conflicts we play out during arguments, breakups, and
divorces are the result of spinning back and forth between our Child
and Adult Substance Shields. Unfortunately, until we gain more command over which shield we are "in," our sexual expressions stay mired
in childish emotions, and we become stressed with insecurity about the
future.

The Spirit Shields

The Substance Shields are relatively easy to picture, probably because
we spend a lot of time bouncing back and forth between them. The
Substance Shields contain everything mortal about us; all the stories,
Light and Dark Arrows, and memories we acquired growing up. The
two spheres pictured orbiting to the left and right sides, however, are
less familiar. They rotate on the East-West axis, and they keep us in the
present moment.

Whereas the Substance Shields are rooted in time, the Spirit Shields
are timeless.

While our Substance Shields collect both positive and negative memories, the Spirit Shields know nothing of past wounding or harm; they
contain only pure potential and presence. The East-West Spirit Shields are
the opposite of our gender, whereas the North-South Substance Shields
are the same gender as our bodies. So, for example, a woman's Child
Substance Shield is referred to as her Little Girl, while her Spirit Shield

contains the energetic of a young boy. Her North Substance Shield is an Adult Woman. Her West Spirit Shield carries the spirit of an Adult Man. The reverse is true for men.[3]

While this may seem complicated, we actually experience these shields all the time. Our Spirit Shields rotate to the front whenever we are completely present and whenever we feel sexy and passionate. When a man needs courage and indomitable will, the Child Spirit Shield (his inner spirit young girl) comes forward. When a woman is in pure action, let's say in the middle of great orgasm, her Adult Spirit Shield spins in front. Whenever we need courage to jump into action because we want to learn and grow, we can call upon our Spirit Shields for help. Quodoushka trainings include many practical techniques to become more familiar with these shields.

Finally, in the center of our luminosity, around the waist, we have what is called our Elder Shield. This is the part of us that is like a wise inner grandmother and grandfather. We can feel the presence of our Elder Shield whenever we act with compassion, generosity, honesty, and wisdom.

WHAT HAPPENS
DURING HIGH-LEVEL ORGASMS

Shamans and Twisted Hairs, who first developed the process of *gleaning*, observed a number of fascinating things. Gleaning is a shamanic term used to describe the ability to perceive, interpret, and measure the changing configurations of light within the aura of anything. The shamans saw that the shapes of the luminous auras of minerals, animals, and plants are different from those of humans. They also observed several interesting things happening to the human luminosity when we have sex. In the same way steam rises above something hot and takes different shapes, they observed the human luminosity rise above the body during high levels of orgasm. When making love, have you ever experienced reaching a place where you could not tell where you ended and your partner began? Have you ever seen the physical features of your lover's face change during intense passion?

THUNDER STRIKES:
IMAGINATION BECOMES REAL

It's not just your imagination. When you change your physical appearance during high-level orgasms, and your lover's face seems to change, or you feel as if you are dissolving in pure light, something is happening to the luminosity: you will experience the opposite gender of your shields.

To gain energy from these experiences, however, you must be able to concentrate your awareness and focus your intent toward the light. In other words, you must learn how to bundle the Fiber Filaments in specific configurations. This is not easy to do in the middle of an orgasm. When you become natural in your rhythmic expression within high-level orgasms, and hold an intention to extend your luminosity, you reestablish your connecting link to Great Spirit's free will. You connect with your original nature and become a cell of Great Spirit's intent.

To understand the shamanic experience, you must be connected to the spiritual sexual energy and understand that you are going through seven dimensions. You actually travel out of your body through different dimensions every night, but you forget what you see. When you dream at night, part of you is here in bed in the third dimension, while another part, called the Dream Mind Body, travels in the fifth dimension.

Besides sleeping and dreaming, there is, however, an even more powerful way to travel in the Dream Mind Body. When you have a fourth- or fifth-level orgasm, you can go into other dimensions and return with knowledge. Those who travel with clear memory are called Journeyers, Travelers, and Twisted Hairs. They travel in the Dream Mind Body willfully and deliberately through spiritual sexual magic. This is considered the anchor of all shamanic practice. It's also called Dreaming of the Nagual.

Through the following practices, you can begin to mutually heighten feelings of pleasure. To do this, you must have ways to perceive more of what is actually occurring when you are making love.

SEXUAL HEALING PRACTICES

◎ Chakra Balancing and Reading

This process is a healing technique that balances the chakras and promotes harmonious circulation of energy through the body. It is used to enhance tender feelings of connection and brings vitality to the chakras. Decide who would like to receive first, and then once you have balanced each other's chakras, switch places. You can create a cozy atmosphere together and sensuously undress for each other. It usually takes about half an hour for each person.

Step One

Giver: Sit on the left side beside the receiver, who is lying down. Take your left hand (Spirit Eye), lift the knee of the receiver, and connect the palm with your partner's left foot (Karma Eye.) This will allow for a deep connection and will facilitate the chakra reading that you will be doing as a part of this exercise.

Leave your right hand free to reach all the chakras (make sure you are both comfortable). When balancing the chakras, you will be enhancing the natural rotation in its appropriate direction. Each chakra rotates either clockwise or counterclockwise. An easy way to remember the difference for men and women is that for women, the odd-numbered chakras rotate counterclockwise and the even-numbered ones rotate clockwise. Thus for men, the first chakra spins clockwise; for women, it spins counterclockwise.

Chakra balancing can be done with a finger or with a crystal held an inch or two above each chakra. Pointing a crystal over the chakra, make at least twenty-one spins in the appropriate direction. Using a finger, place the third finger over the index finger, point it toward and above the chakra, and swirl your hand at the wrist to create small circles about three or four inches in diameter.

After the twenty-first spin, lightly tap the index finger on the skin over the chakra for an instant and then lift your finger or the crystal a quarter-inch away from the body. So, for example, if you were at the third chakra, you would lightly touch the navel. This grounds the energy.

As you rotate each chakra, beginning with the 1st and ending with the 7th, imagine pulling energy in through the top of your head with each inhalation and then breathing this fire energy out through your arm and finger into your partner's chakra with each exhalation. Try using your Fiber Filaments to enhance your sensitivity.

Receiver: Relax and lie quietly and feel whatever you feel.

Step Two

Giver: Now that the chakras are spinning with vitality and you have finished the rotation, "read" the images that appear in connection with each chakra. They give insight into your partner's current physical, emotional, mental, or spiritual condition.

Adjust your position to sit comfortably, holding the receiver's right foot with the left hand while still being able to reach each chakra. You will probably need to bend the receiver's leg at the knee.

Then place the palm of your right hand above the chakra and let an image come to your mind. Briefly relate this image to your partner. Say the very first picture, feeling, thought, sound, or color that comes to mind. For example, you might say, "Green field," or the title of a song that comes to you. Do not judge this; simply say the first thing that appears. It does not have to make sense to you, but it may be very important for your partner. It may tell him or her something valuable to help keep the chakra energies flowing.

When you have completed all seven chakras, switch positions.

◎ Chakra-Merging Exercise

Chakra merging helps partners align and energize their chakras and thus creates a wonderful sense of connection and oneness. It is an excellent way to enhance intimacy before making love, and it can also be a great way to connect if for some reason you do not wish to have intercourse or other forms of sex. Although we say female and male partner here for the sake of describing two partners, women or men can easily practice chakra merging with marvelous results.

Step One

Male Partner: Sit on a cushion cross-legged.

Female Partner: Sit on top of the male partner, placing your legs around his torso with the soles of your feet touching each other. This will place all your chakras together. If you know each other well, you can place the man's tipili upright between you. You can also place his tipili between the outer lips of your tupuli, if you are comfortable doing so.

Male Partner: Place your hands on either side of the woman's buttocks toward the back and put gentle pressure there.

Once you are comfortable, begin by breathing naturally together and uniting the timing of your breath before you start merging chakras.

Female Partner: Put your arms around your partner. Place your left palm on the man's back at the height of his heart chakra, and your right palm where his shoulder meets his neck.

Lead the chakra merging with the timing of your breath and contractions.

Male Partner: Become receptive and follow her timing. If you lose the timing, simply return to the speed and rhythm of her breath.

Next, both partners take in a deep breath. With the inhalation, focus on and "breathe into" your first chakra as if you are taking in air through your genitals. Hold your breath while you contract and relax your perineum muscles about seven times. At the same time, concentrate your energy from your own first chakra into your partner's. Then, exhale gently into each other's right ears. You are drawing the energy inward and upward, similar to doing Kegel exercises.

Repeat breathing and contracting at the first chakra until there is a feeling of warm energy flow and connection between both of your first chakras. Repeat inhaling, contracting, exhaling, and relaxing at the first chakra at least five times. The number of times is not important; feeling sensations of heat or energy around the genitals is what matters.

Then, when the woman decides, bring your attention to the second chakra. Imagine energy and air flowing between your second chakras below the navel. Continue on to the third, fourth, fifth, and sixth chakras until the energy rises through your bodies and lifts up to your crown chakras at the top of your heads.

Helpful hints

- The female partner presses or taps on her partner's back to the timing of her contractions, so that he can contract and breathe at the same speed. The male partner allows himself to become so receptive that he completely surrenders to his partner's breath and movements.

- When the female partner feels it is time to move on to the next chakra, whisper the number of that chakra gently into the male partner's ear, and then both of you shift attention to the next chakra.

- If the seated position is uncomfortable, you can also practice chakra merging by lying on your sides while entwining your legs together. The chakras align in the same manner through the central channel of your bodies. If there is a great height difference, what's most important is keeping the first chakras together as best you can.

- Try out different timing of inward breaths and contractions, fast or slow, and see which suits you both best. You can bring wonderful sensuality to this exercise by adding a gentle back-and-forth pelvic rocking motion in time with your contractions.

- Typically, once you feel a sense of energy or heat around your navels at the third chakras, breath and movements accelerate. It may take you several tries to feel the energy reach the navel, but when it does, the rest will come quickly. When you reach the fourth chakra, there is often a tremendous rush of intimacy as your heart energies merge. Keep going to the fifth chakra at the throat. Here, partners often moan or make passionate sounds, and often your heads will arch backward because the energy wants to move through the mouth. Sometimes when you reach the sixth chakra at the brow center, you may wish to place your foreheads together. Continue to bring the energy upward. If you lose the sensation, or get out of sync, simply focus again on the first chakra for a few moments and bring the energy up again through each chakra. Once you reach the sixth chakra at the brow, you will feel a strong surge of energy move through your head. It is as if you are having an orgasm, and actually you are, only it's an energy orgasm. Frequently, couples arch backward and make sounds similar to those during genitally focused orgasms. Sometimes this feels so good you will want to do it again. If this happens, and you feel as if you have entered an ongoing loop of sexual energy, you have succeeded in having a high-level orgasmic experience.

• Try not to compare chakra merging to genitally focused sex; it is wonderfully different. Enjoy being intimate afterward in any way you like.

THE ART OF SELF-PLEASURING

It could be said that our first sexual experience is with ourselves. It is well documented that infants in the womb rub their own genitals. Yet there is a long history of negative associations connected with masturbation. The word *masturbate* was first recorded in 1857. It's derived from the Latin word *manstrupare*. *Turbare* means "to stir up," *manu* means "hand," and *stupare* means "to defile (oneself)."

More recently, in 1994 the U.S. surgeon general, Jocelyn Elders, was fired after a controversial reply to a question at a United Nations conference. She was asked whether masturbation would be appropriate to promote as a means of preventing young people from engaging in riskier forms of sexual activity. She replied, "I think that it is part of human sexuality, and perhaps it should be taught."

Quodoushka uses the phrase *self-pleasuring* as a way to encode an entirely different message and introduces the Self or Heart-Pleasuring Exercise as a method to increase the intensity of orgasmic pleasure. Heart Pleasuring is a solo practice that helps connect our sexual feelings with our heart. Instead of feeling hurried with shame or guilt, self-pleasuring can be used as one way to gain greater control with the timing of ejaculations. When it is practiced with a celebratory attitude that says, "I do deserve pleasure," the Heart-Pleasuring Exercise restores our primal sexual connection with our own body. It does away with unnecessary negative feelings we may unconsciously carry about allowing ourselves pleasure. It is also an excellent way to increase libido and brings more heart-centered feelings into our lovemaking.

This exercise combines the use of self-pleasuring with energy focus on the chakras.

For the best results, practice regularly on your own about three times per week for at least three months.

◎ Self-Pleasuring Exercise

- Begin to self-pleasure in your favorite way (manually, vibrator, running water, etc.).
- As you continue to self-pleasure, begin to focus your energy and intent on the first chakra.
- With your inhalation, imagine pulling the energy into your first chakra; and as you exhale, imagine this energy expanding into your genitals.
- Continue self-pleasuring as you focus on the first chakra until it feels very "full."
- Next, move your awareness to the second chakra below the navel, and repeat the same process, inhaling and pulling the energy into the second chakra and exhaling as you allow energy to expand within the second chakra.
- As each chakra becomes "full" and you feel the energy is rising, move your awareness to the next chakra. When you reach the heart chakra, create a large loop of energy from the first chakra to the heart and back to the first.
- As you become more excited, increase the pace of your breathing. With your inhalation, pull the energy up to the fourth chakra, and with your exhalation, send it out the fourth down to the first again.
- Once you begin to feel sensations around your heart, bring yourself

almost to the point of orgasm. But right before you come, just before you would have gone over the edge, completely relax.

Do this three times, bringing yourself to the brink of an orgasm, but instead, totally relax your entire body. At this point, focus all your energy into your heart chakra. On the fourth time, allow the orgasm to explode while you again focus all your energy on your heart chakra. Imagine radiant warmth emanating from your heart.

CONTINUING PLEASURE

As you practice bringing yourself to the brink and relaxing, it will soon cease to be an exercise. You will notice several wonderful things: your orgasms become more intense, and you will find yourself luxuriating in intense sexual energy with far greater presence.

Try to avoid being too rigid about counting the number of times you approach climax. Sometimes you will only manage to delay two orgasms. Keep in mind that if it becomes a chore, then the effects are not as strong. You are resculpting pleasure back into your body, and it's meant to be arousing and fun.

Once you get the hang of this, you can also use this technique for mutual merging during intercourse. Through genital stimulation of intercourse, bring yourselves almost to the point of orgasm three times. On the fourth time, focus the energy on your fourth chakras and feel the orgasmic release through your hearts. Imagine radiant warmth joining you together as one.

Although the Fire Breath is only taught to students with personal guidance from a qualified Quodoushka instructor, the following story of how Thunder Strikes learned this technique will give you valuable insights into the nature of this practice.

The Fire Breath

The Fire Breath is actually a warrior's technique of discipline taught to me by my clan uncles when I was a young boy. I learned how to breathe when I was stalking, tracking, and hunting in the woods. Something happens when you are completely alone with no other humans around; if you learn to breathe properly, you drop into expanded states where you can feel, sense, and align with everything around you. To fully connect with prey, you must be able to breathe with them instead of being in your own world. This creates a totally different kind of connection, and the same thing is true when you are with a lover.

The Fire Breath is the centering breath that puts you in touch with nature. It teaches you to stop trying to be superior to other things around you. It's a harmony of nature breath that induces a natural orgasmic response. If you observe cetaceans, especially dolphins, you will see they are in a state of constant orgasmic energy. They do not have body orgasms the way we do, but they're always in an orgasmic state. Since your body is inside your mind, the Fire Breath teaches you to stay in the natural orgiastic state with nature, and therefore you can be more natural when you are with another, regardless of your sexual preferences. This is actually our natural state, but we block it all the time.

THUNDER STRIKES

The technique of Fire Breathing recalibrates your internal organs by circulating vital orgasmic energy throughout the entire body. With practice, you can have a full-body orgasm that feels as if you are climaxing with a release similar to, yet quite different from, a genital orgasm. The Fire Breath uses a combination of breath and muscle control to bring the flow of energy up through the chakras to produce a powerful orgasmic experience. Unlike our usual orgasms, which are genitally localized, the Fire Breath generates more of a "soul orgasm" in which the whole body is excited in multiple waves of sensation. Rather than a short peak-and-release, vibrating pleasure comes in prolonged surges and plateaus of extended ecstasy lasting a few minutes to several hours.

Typically, following the Fire Breath's peak, you will feel connected to everything in the same way you might after having a high-level orgasm. It is amazing, and perhaps at first disconcerting, to have the same expanded feelings without even touching your genitals. For men, most often there is no erection, and for women, quivers move from the top of the head to the tips of the toes. Although the benefits are great, because we are not used to breathing in this manner, practicing the Fire Breath on your own can bring up intense emotional and physical responses that you may not understand how to deal with. It is best therefore to practice the Chakra Balancing and Chakra Merging techniques first, before receiving instructions on the Fire Breath from a qualified Quodushka teacher who can guide you in mastering this technique.

13

The Eight Lovers' Masks

EXPANDING YOUR EROTIC PERSONA

Nothing is more important for your erotic life than being an interesting and, at times, unpredictable lover. Bringing new ideas into the bedroom, or better yet, venturing beyond familiar territory is the best way to ward off relationship monotony. Just as the finest dish in the world may have tasted incredible that first time, it gets bland if it's served too often. While it is possible to get by with sex as you know it, it's the spice you bring to the table that makes your partner want you more.

This wheel brings out your personality as a lover and inspires you to try sexual things you may have always wanted to do. If you've ever had an extended lull, chances are you were giving only one or two of the Lovers' Masks airtime in your sex life. How would you like to be approached by an adventurer full of sensuous wonder? Or get into the carnal sensations of the body in a spree of spontaneous fun? Then shift gears, and see how easily you can change direction to have more of the kind of sexual intimacy you deserve.

It is said, whether we are aware of it or not, we are always wearing a Lover's Mask. As we cruise though our days, we may don the mask of an entrepreneur, a secretary, or a hairdresser, but underneath whatever outfit we wear in the world, we are lovers seeking expression. Even if you are walking around in sweatpants and sex is the furthest thing from your mind, you are still broadcasting something about your sexual persona. The question is: are you hiding behind an unconscious mask and sending signals that prevent you from having sex? Are there parts of you that long to come out and play?

Shamanic traditions have always used masks in tribal celebrations because they give the dancer permission to unleash and display unusual, eccentric things. Wearing a mask lets us transcend the ordinary to expose our inner yearnings. When we choose to play sexually within a Lover's Mask, we can let go of inhibitions and be bolder. We have the chance to show neglected sides of ourselves and delve into forgotten feelings of pleasure. Expanding your sexuality to include several directions on this wheel not only adds juice to your love life, each mask shows you how to enchant your partner in different ways.

There is no one way to play any of these Lovers' Masks. Once you understand the healing quality of each direction, the only limitation is your imagination. Use the following stories as starting points to create your own scenarios and have fun making your lover's journey full of surprise, passion, or maybe, a leap into total surrender.

SOUTH

The Shy, Curious Lover's Mask

That Girl in the Pink Dress

I had just returned from an unusual shopping fling one afternoon when my boyfriend came over for lunch. While he was in the kitchen, I decided to try on my new outfit. You could see the full-length mirror in my bedroom from the kitchen, so he was watching me change. I had been to Kmart to shop for something I never in my wildest dreams thought I would ever wear: a pink frilly dress with a white lace collar. It was a size twelve I bought in the

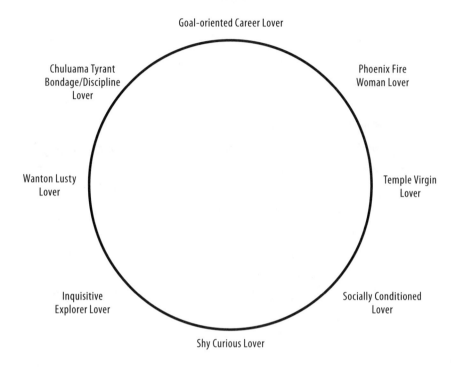

Fig. 13.1. The Lovers' Masks

children's department. I altered it a bit by cutting out the inner lining so you could see my breasts through the pink bodice, and of course you could see right through the tiny skirt at the bottom too. I was admiring myself in the mirror and reveling in the fact that I actually fit into something a girl would wear. But when I looked at my reflection, I got quite a lovely shock: I saw my boyfriend standing behind me with a huge grin and a huge hard-on.

The rush was unbelievable. I felt so young and giddy standing there in that pink lacey dress with his hard-on staring at me in the mirror. I couldn't believe he was so turned on! Needless to say, that afternoon, as he lifted me onto the bed, peeling back the pink folds over my thighs, I became a woman.

But there's more to the story, about how this Lover's Mask was unusually healing for me. All my life I had been shy about my small breasts. I compared them to my sister's and others' who had what I thought were more womanly breasts. I saw the way men adore breasts, and I always felt mine were too small to arouse much interest.

That afternoon, however, everything about the way I felt about my breasts changed. Perhaps it was the adventure of buying a pink dress that made me feel incredibly innocent and shy. While we were sprawled on the bed, holding and caressing each other, I mentioned the way I felt about my breasts. For some reason, this produced another rousing round of passion. Through his kisses he told me how much he loved my breasts; he caressed them and tasted them for what seemed an eternity. I had no idea my shyness could be so allur- ing. I felt completely beautiful.

Since then, once in a while, whenever I am feeling too serious, I deliber- ately step into a much softer, sweeter, and more vulnerable part of myself. I may not fit into that dress anymore, but there are plenty of ways to get back in touch with the lovely girl inside me. I like to get in the mood by doing some- thing fun. What amazes me is that not only do I like the curious, playful side of myself; it never fails to elicit a fantastic response.

AMARA

The curious child that lives inside is one of the most alluring and attractive facets of our lover's persona. Seen in this way, feeling shy or reluctant about making love can be extremely endearing, especially if it is not your normal role. The Shy, Curious Mask is also the part of us that loves being playful. There's nothing more healing than to be frivolous or rowdy from time to time. Whenever we are full of trust and innocence, we are tapping into the healing energies of this mask.

Being shy or curious is not about acting coy or clever the way little girls and boys can get. The dark side is to act childish, withholding sex or using it to get what you want. Children are not mature enough to have sex, and childish manipulations have no place in adult sexual behavior. Pretending that someone is a child or treating someone like a child is the exact opposite of this mask's intent.

On the light side, you can be rambunctious or tentative in the begin- ning of foreplay. If you need to get the ball rolling and want to let go of some stress, try casually flirting, turning on the power of the curious boy or girl who loves getting attention. Then, as the things get cooking, become the sensuous man or woman ready for some mature sexy passion.

SOUTHWEST

The Adventurer/Explorer Lover's Mask

Charlene's Sailboat Bliss

My husband and I were married for eleven years, and you can be sure nothing like this had ever happened, even in the beginning of our relationship. He rented a big sailboat for my birthday in San Diego for the weekend. On the first night, we started to kiss on the deck under the stars and reminisce about past birthdays together. He always liked to surprise me with things, but this is the one I will never forget. Since we don't really know how to sail, I was surprised by his plan, and I was already in heaven, but it turns out he had much more in mind. I guess you could say it was sailing of a different kind. He disappeared into the cabin and came back with what looked like fixings for ice cream sundaes. He had bananas and cherries, chocolate sauce and whipped cream, only there were no bowls or spoons to be found. I guess I was the dish that night, because he made a banana split out of me! It was pretty cold, with ice cream melting over my naked body, but I didn't mind when he started licking whipped cream around my private parts. He dribbled chocolate sauce and cherries all over, and of course he saved the banana for the best part . . . To this day, we like to eat banana splits on my birthday, just to remember that glorious, glorious sailboat night.

A Flair for the Dramatic

My girlfriend definitely has a taste for wide-open spaces. Little did I know just how much of a taste. This wasn't something we planned; it was spontaneous, which was the best part of it all. One night my girlfriend insisted we go to the place where she graduated from high school. It was a fantastic outdoor amphitheater for big outdoor concerts. There were thousands of empty seats and a huge stage lit only by moonlight. I couldn't have imagined a more romantic spot. That night, much to my delight, there was not a soul in sight. I was planning to take her on an evening picnic with wine in a quiet place on the hill in the back, but she was dying to walk on the stage. So we took our bottle and glasses and went down to have a look. I was singing, listening to the echoes flying out over the seats, when she started to unbutton my shirt. I looked around to see if anyone was there, but pretty soon we were only thinking of each other. It was incredible, making love on center stage. It felt like we had an audience of gods. It was magnificent, and totally unexpected. Fortunately, I have the rest of my life to savor that memory.

JERRY

Strangers at a Hotel

It had been a long time since my partner and I had done anything out of the ordinary, and to tell you the truth, we were in a kind of rut sexually. We thought we would try role-playing, so one night we planned an elaborate evening of intrigue and mystery. We arranged to meet at a crowded bar on a Saturday, only we decided to be strangers for the night. I dressed in my best Brooks Brothers suit with a black fedora, and my wife was dressed to the hilt too. We drove in separate cars and flirted with other people for a while, but we kept sending furtive glances to each other from across the room. I made up a new identity, telling people I had grown up in a foster home and had just returned from China from a business trip that was worth my weight in gold. I overheard my wife, and I could tell by the look on her face that she was concocting a fantastic ruse too. It was great pretending we were other people, and I couldn't wait to hear what she was conjuring up. Finally, I told the bartender to buy the lovely lady at the end of the bar a drink. (I knew what she liked, but ordered something else instead.) She graciously accepted and gave a little note to the bartender to give to me. It said, "Would you care to join me?"

I sauntered over to her feeling like a single man again and asked her where she was from. She was a painter on retreat preparing for an exhibition. "And what kind of pictures do you paint?" I asked, trying to sound suave with my fake accent. "Well, actually," she said, "my favorite subject is male nudes, and I am looking for my next model. Interested?"

That was my cue. I hired a suite and began "posing" for my wife. It was hilarious at times, but excellent fun. We weren't perfect at the game, but I think she loved me more for trying. I had never been looked at as an object of art, and it was actually quite exciting. She made me wait for what seemed like forever. It was wonderful to feel wanted again. I never imagined being creative like that could be such an amazing turn-on. We made love with more passion than we had for years. Since then, whenever the embers are burning low, I call her Madame and she calls me Sir Mathias, and we laugh about that fantastic night.

MARY AND RICHARD

This mask is about feeling like you can find fresh territory to explore no matter how many times you have made love before. Whenever you are trying out something new, making love in unusual places, and most of all, being spontaneous, you are wearing the Adventurer/Explorer's Lover's Mask. It is not always easy to do, and our adventures do not always work out perfectly, but in the end, the pleasure that comes from daring to step into the unknown sides of ourselves makes the risks worth taking. The more you make creativity a hallmark of your lover's persona, always on the lookout for a little something new to give, the more enduring and sexy your love life will become.

The dark side of this mask is when the need for novelty becomes excessive, and everyday sexual interest is not enough. Being an Explorer means to notice when you are bored and then finding something new to stir the mystery and magic between you. Any relationship can get sleepy from time to time, and everyone loves to be surprised. Yet, while doing something novel is exciting—like secretly arranging a private masseuse for your honey—giving small, unexpected gestures of affection is equally wonderful. Before going away on a trip, try leaving little love notes in pockets, cupboards, and inside books you know will be read while you are away. You may be the one surprised when you return.

WEST

The Lusty, Passionate Lover's Mask

The Striptease

I was the kind of guy who was petrified to ask a girl to dance, and I am not exactly the most outgoing type of person. One evening, however, a few of my myths got flipped upside down. I had been on only three or four dates with a new girlfriend. I thought things were going smoothly enough, and although I was ready and hoping for a bit more, I wasn't in any hurry to be sexual. I guess maybe she thought I wasn't interested, but that was not the case at all.

Anyway, I think she was feeling things could get a little hotter between us, because one night, out of the blue, she asked me to strip for her. I thought only men liked to watch strippers, and that male strippers were for gay men. I had no idea women liked that sort of thing. Well, at first I flat-out refused, but she wouldn't take no for an answer. She started begging me in such a totally seductive way. How could I say no? The truth is, I was petrified, but I used that fear of mine, closed my eyes, listened to the sexy music she turned on, and just started slowly, really slowly, taking off my clothes for her. It wasn't fancy, mind you, but she seemed to like it a lot. I think I did it for her because she kept looking in my eyes with such a pleading smile, and my tech-nique didn't seem to matter. All I can say is that it was the best date I ever had. The truth is, I felt like a king showing off for her, and it felt really good. With some practice, I think I could even get good at this!

BRUCE

To get the juices rolling for sex, one of the common ways to play the Wanton Lover's Mask is to dress in sexy lingerie. This is the lusty part of us that revels in naked bodies, kissing, licking, and sucking, and that welcomes the passion of pure physical sex. Anytime we openly let our sexual hungers be seen, we are wearing this mask.

In the beginning of courtship, our wanton, lusty self is alive and well, but as time goes by, it is sometimes the most difficult part of our lover's persona to access. The dark side of this mask is when you become overly aggressive and self-absorbed about sex. Focusing on the physical aspects alone, bypassing sensuous touch and intimate conversation, it turns dark when it's all about getting off and conquest is the overriding motivation.

While being passionate as a lover may not be something as easy to turn on as a light, there are plenty of ways to ensure the lusty side of you comes out for a romp. As much as we may enjoy cuddling and talking about sex, there are times we need to have intense physical sex. Greeting your partner in a slinky gown ready for a quickie when he comes home from work or making dinner wearing a skimpy apron works like a charm. To get in the mood for a hot night, try wearing silk panties underneath a business suit and see what it does for your career. It may not land the deal, but who knows, the smile on your face every time you feel that luxurious tug against your body may turn a few heads your way. For gentlemen, try wearing an elegant silk robe, or for the more adventurous, perhaps a bare chest, a cowboy hat, and great jeans with the zipper open will do the trick.

NORTHWEST

The Mistress/Master—Submissive Lover's Mask

The Mistress Dom

I am a businesswoman with a lot of authority. I have several people working for me, and I guess you could say I have things under control. I take care of

the kids and the house in addition to having a tight-laced, high-paced career.
My private sex life, however, is the place where I like to let go of it all. On
the one hand, I like to be "on top," but in reality, I am secretly submissive.
Sometimes, I like my man to wear nylons so that I can see everything he has
wrapped up like a present for me. First, I want him to do exactly as I say, but
then, somewhere in the middle, when he gets turned on and starts feeling his
power, I become soft and delicate for him. The tables turn, and now it's me
who is wearing a collar and blindfold, doing as I am told. I like being taken
by him, and I want him to give me everything he's got, usually until he can't
move anymore. The kind of tenderness that comes out from both of us is like
food for my soul. He is utterly sensitive to me, and never crosses the line with
any kind of pain. Although I usually play the submissive, once in a while I like
to play the mistress too.

BELLA

In a certain sense, we play this mask all the time. It's not that we walk around wearing the commonly known emblems—leather garb, blindfolds, or restraints. It's that we often play inside the role of being the "top" or "bottom" in our everyday lives. In the language of this Lover's Mask, depending on the situation, we are either more dominant or more submissive. In arenas where we have expertise, we may be a "dom," and in other areas we may be a "sub" and like to follow. Generally, we gravitate toward one side or the other. It is also called the Tyrant's Lover's Mask because if we are overly controlling or too submissive, the role becomes oppressive.

Choosing to play this Lover's Mask in your private sex life gives you the opportunity to switch the role you normally play in life. It lets you explore feelings of surrender or of masterful leadership. If you have an intense life with complex responsibilities, surrendering into a submissive sexual place provides tremendous relief. On the other hand, if you are often under the direction of others, becoming the mistress or the master of the bedroom can be incredibly stimulating. Because these sexual dynamics are so powerful, and they bring out intense and sometimes unexpected responses, when you step into the sexual territory with this Lover's Mask, you must always exercise exceptional care.

Seen in this way, this Lover's Mask can be one of the most powerful healing expressions on the wheel. The challenge of learning to be the mistress or master who leads the scenario, or the submissive who succumbs to his or her feelings of pleasure, can bring tremendous passion into your sex play, especially if you have never tried this before. To fully let go in ecstasy, however, we need to trust our partner completely. Thus, the first rule to remember when playing the Northwest mask is to share this only with someone you feel entirely comfortable with.

The Secret to Being the Mistress or Master of Pleasure

As the mistress or master, your primary focus is on is the delicacy and vulnerability of your partner. When you are playing the "top," you are creating a space for your lover to relinquish control. Keep in mind that you are giving permission for him or her to feel sensations and emotions that long to come out. You must at all times determine to take care of your lover's physical body, because you are fully responsible for his or her safety.

The secret to being a great "dom" is to have one and only one thing on your mind: *your partner's pleasure.* In fact, while it may seem as if you are leading, in reality, everything you do is dictated by your lover's acute desire for greater erotic sensation. When you get good at seeing what your lover really likes, you might give just a tease and then make him or her plead for more.

Rules for Playing Safely on the Edges of Ecstasy

Make several agreements before you start. To create a place to safely explore, before you step into being a master or submissive, agree on a code word that means stop. Since unpredictable things may occur, and unfamiliar feelings may surface, you should always start by creating a code word that means stop everything immediately. It's best to use something other than "Stop," because this word may already be used in the course of your lovemaking. Your code word should be a simple, out-of-context word, such as "Pineapple." If "Pineapple" is spoken, drop whatever you are doing right away and then talk about what you are experiencing. It is also suggested you agree beforehand on a time limit for playing within these roles.

Causing physical pain, such as bruising, cutting, or asphyxiation, is outside the boundaries of this mask. The intent is to tease with pleasure and to heighten feelings of anticipation. In my opinion, physical pain has no place in a healthy sexual relationship. There is never a need to cause or use a threat of physical or emotional injury in any way. As you are being teased into a stupor of sheer joy, and are giving yourself permission to surrender, never, under any circumstances, submit to any physical or emotional harm whatsoever. Quodoushka promotes only light explorations into the dynamics of pleasure and views pain as contrary to this mask's intent.

The Secret of Being Submissive

For whatever reasons, it is really a challenge to admit how much we want sexual pleasure. The secret to being a great submissive is to drop your inhibitions and admit how badly you want something. Being submissive does not mean agreeing to let someone do what ever he or she wants to do. It means creating the conditions for your safety, and then letting go to feel pleasure freely inside agreed-upon boundaries. Actual humiliation or putting each other down is not a part of this mask's intention.

Therefore, agree on the kinds of things you will use to tease each other. For example, you may choose a leather whip, silk restraints, feathers, or a blindfold. (The brisk sweep of a leather whip or being tied to a bedpost can be exhilarating—if you know what you are doing.) Make sure you know how to use these things, and if you are not sure, test them out beforehand, or research online about how to use them safely. If this is new territory, while it may seem to limit the surprise, it is necessary to discuss all details of your Northwest Lover's Mask before you start.

The dark side of this Lover's Mask, in addition to taking things too far and causing pain, is to be obsessive with its use. Being the master or mistress, or a love slave longing to be seduced, can be thrilling. Once you get a taste of the energy it generates, the extreme buzz can become addictive. It may be tempting to return to the same roles again and again to get off on feelings of power or surrender, but using any one of these Lover's Masks all the time will create an imbalance in your relationship. Try changing roles to experience what each side feels like. When used sparingly, with perhaps a blindfold and feathers for an occasional change rather than as your main menu, these powerful dynamics can bring you into unforgettably deep spaces of exquisite sexual passion.

NORTH

The Career- or Goal-Oriented Lover's Mask

We are wearing a Career- or Goal-Oriented Lover's Mask whenever we make a clear agreement about the value of sex. The sexual mores of any society assess the worth, price, and value placed upon various aspects of sex. While, on the one hand, it is impossible to calculate the cost of sexual love, and we like to think sex is a priceless, mysterious commodity, the reality is that we use this Lover's Mask all the time. In one sense, a marriage is a sexual contract that places value on fidelity. The agreement to have sex a certain number of times per week, or an agreement to be sexual for a limited time, are examples of using a Goal-Oriented Lover's Mask.

In various societies during different eras, sexual favors have been highly valued. Certain Buddhist and Hindu philosophical systems created tantric schools of thought with the understanding that sex, as a basic and powerful desire experienced by all humans, could be utilized as a way of achieving enlightenment. Tantric traditions spread throughout Asia, Indonesia, and Japan and created the traditions of tantrikas, courtesans, and geisha, who were often well paid for their sexual expertise. For thousands of years, until the Communist regime outlawed the custom of multiple wives in China, the social status and sexual expectations of women were clearly delineated through various legal contracts. Thai society has its own unique set of sexual mores. The polygamist tradition of having *mia noi* (mistresses) is still practiced among the wealthier elites.

While prostitution is officially illegal in Thailand, prosecution is rarely enforced, and the sex trade generates billions of dollars per year.

Consequently, visiting a paid mistress is not uncommon. Many Thai women believe the existence of paid mistresses actively reduces the incidence of rape. Nonetheless, the degrading, humiliating subjugation of women and minors in slave trades, Hollywood deals, or in any situation where men or woman are coerced into selling sex are examples of the dark side of this Lover's Mask.

Today in New Zealand, prostitution laws are some of the most liberal in the world, and it is one of the few countries where brothels are legal. Exchanging money for sex is also legal in certain jurisdictions in the Netherlands, Australia, Germany, and Las Vegas, Nevada. What interests us here, however, is how we can use the Career- or Goal-Oriented Lover's Mask to create clear, conscious, and empowering sexual agreements in our own lives.

Lisa: Where to Turn for Sex

Living without sex for over two years was simply unacceptable. I tried going to bars and singles parties and finally joined an Internet dating service, but I couldn't find Mr. Right. After going on one too many unsuccessful dates, while I still wanted to find that special person to spend the rest of my life with, I really needed to make love. I decided that waiting this long was not working for me. Then one day I was having lunch with a friend I had known for years, but never considered as a sexual partner. When I casually brought up the idea of having sex, he was a bit surprised. I explained that I wasn't looking for a relationship with him and wondered if he would be open to an occasional encounter.

It was a new idea for both of us. My main fear was, what if he got attached and wanted more?' Or, what if I wanted more once we had sex? We talked about our concerns for several hours as the idea settled in. We knew things were bound to change once sex was brought into our friendship, and so we agreed to be honest about feelings we couldn't predict. Interestingly, the conversation made me feel more attracted to him. I had never talked to someone in such detail, bringing up possible problems before making love! We agreed to limit our rendezvous to a once-a-week date, to talk on the phone during the week, and to have another conversation in a month to see how this was working.

The sex we shared was not the most passionate sex I have ever had, but it was precious. He knew I was still looking for a life partner. After a few months I met someone I wanted to date more intimately, and so we decided to end our special dates. My friend was happy for me, and I will always be grateful for what we shared. In some way, I feel that opening myself to him sexually freed up feelings that were buried inside for far too long. I think our sex dates paved the way for my new relationship.

NORTHEAST

Phoenix Fireman/Firewoman Lover's Mask

Everything Had to Change

My wife went through almost a year of chemotherapy and radiation treatments for cancer. Needless to say, our once-happy sex life changed completely, and we weren't sure we could ever recover. It was heartbreaking watching her going through so much pain and feeling sick most of the time. Sex the way we knew it was out of the question, and she did not feel the least bit sexy during those many months. It was hard for me too, because I didn't feel like having sex much either; but the energy was building up inside, and I needed to find something else to do with it.

So I decided to learn everything I could about alternate ways to be sexual. It was surprising how much hope this gave both of us. I shared everything I found with her; I read books and got videos on sensuous touch, and really erotic things like anal massage and extended orgasms. I learned about the Fire Breath and Self-Pleasuring. I studied sexual anatomy and everything I could get my hands on about female desire. I know my wife saw how seriously

I was studying these things, and it made her feel like I was waiting for her, and I was. At first it was a little strange just reading and looking at all these things, but I made up my mind we were going to win. I let her know that whatever it took, however I needed to change, and whatever I needed to learn, we were going to become even better lovers. I think it gave her a reason to get well.

Before her treatments, sex was fantastic, and I didn't feel the need to know much more. Afterward, once she recovered, everything was different, and I am glad to say we found out how to enjoy sex in ways we probably would never have looked into. For the first months, I just lovingly held her without any expectations at all. I took care of my own needs privately, and I let her know I was fine. I never tried to arouse her, and I waited for her to make the first move, whenever she was ready. Then one morning she started to stroke my penis. Even then I tried to stay relatively calm so there was no pressure to go further—I knew she was still weak, and I wanted her to know she had all the time in the world, and that I wasn't going anywhere. Looking back, I think that's the most important thing—that I was right there and that there was no hurry at all. What we learned through my wife's illness, especially about patience, will always be there, and sex for us will never be the same as it was. It really is better now. Does that make me a sexual healer? I don't think so. I just love my wife, and for me there was never a doubt we would find a way.

Jоhn

Whenever you come to your lover with the desire to bring tenderness, kindness, and loving touch, you are wearing a face of the Phoenix Fireman/Firewoman Lover's Mask. This is an aspect of your lover's persona that knows when to initiate sensuous closeness or drop into passionate abandon. It's also the lover's face you wear as a healer.

The path of using this mask to turn lovemaking into profoundly healing experiences begins with learning the nuances and details of your partner's needs. You can use the sexual anatomy teachings as a starting point. As you become intimately familiar with the types and identify your own and your partner's genital anatomy, you will learn the degrees of pressure and positions, as well as the timing of when to slow down or quicken, when to talk sexy, or what kind of sensuous surprises your partner likes. You will not only come to know his or her preferences, you will discover how to masterfully take what he or she likes into intensely fulfilling states of sensuous pleasure.

Assuming the role of a Fireman/Firewoman Lover can be as simple as cajoling your partner, enticing her to open and make love when she is feeling overwhelmed, or helping him totally relax when he is tense and stressed. Or it can be using everything you know to create high-level orgasms. On another level, a man or woman uses the role of Phoenix Fireman/Firewoman Lover's Mask by becoming highly trained in the skills of sexual healing. Understanding the powerful consequences of emotional, mental, physical, and spiritual energies, a Firewoman or Fireman learns to use sexual energy to help restore health and relationships and treat symptoms such as early ejaculations or weakened libido. The Quodoushka training for becoming a Phoenix Firewoman or Fireman takes many years of extensive education and requires ceremonial experiences in the Sweet Medicine Sundance Path.

EAST

Priestess/Priest Lover's Mask

Ceremonial Nights

The whole idea of bringing ceremony into our sex life was new to us. My husband and I always treated sex as something special, but bringing these new ingredients and making a lovemaking ritual of it all took everything to a higher level. My husband makes custom furniture, and one day he brought home a small table he had built and declared it our "sex altar." We carved our names into it the way you scratch initials into a tree. On nights when one of us feels especially horny, we bring out candles, incense, and flowers we arrange just for the occasion. There is one stone we put in the center if we really want to make love. We have an agreement that unless we are sick, if one of us puts the stone in the center, we will have sex within twenty-four hours no matter what. We have done this for over seven years and have never once broken our agreement. I love seeing that stone sitting there, because I know he only puts it there when he truly desires me, and he needs to feel closer. I use it sparingly too, just to keep it special. For some reason, it's better than asking.

There is another wonderful thing about our Ceremonial Nights. We dedicate our orgasms and all our pleasure to be sent where it's needed. Once we put a picture of our son, who was going on a tour of duty in Afghanistan, on the altar. Right before we climaxed into a beautiful reverie, we looked into each other's eyes, saw the picture, and sent our son loving thoughts and prayers. Afterward, we talked about how much we adore him. We believe sex can be a healing force, just like a prayer you might send to someone in need. Somehow, the simple act of lighting our special candles, setting up the altar, and burning the incense makes everything magical. Lovemaking is especially tender, and I look forward to these nights very much.

SHERYL AND DAVE

There is no well-known equivalent to the Temple Priest/Priestess Lover's Mask in our culture, yet whenever you create a love nest and dedicate the energy of your lovemaking to others, you are wearing this mask. Tantric and shamanic practitioners who celebrate sex as a means to enhance visions cultivate unique ways to direct the healing powers of sex. One of the most powerful ways to step into the role of a Temple Priest and Priestess is to consciously bring a child into the world. During lovemaking, you might imagine the qualities of the child you desire to give birth to. To fortify your orgasmic energies, you can create relaxed times to make love, prepare certain healthy foods, and be especially kind toward each other. The Quodoushka tradition provides steps for couples to unite their energies in sexual magical ceremonies to manifest desires of the heart. (See chapter 15.)

SOUTHEAST

The Socially Conditioned Lover's Mask

Rule Number Six

Once a minister of a country was attending an important international diplomatic convention. In the middle of the conference, more than half the members started shouting out slogans when chaos broke loose over some major negotiation. The chairman, who was a resident in the convention's host country, stood up, pounded his gavel, and said to the man instigating the unrest, "Sir, may I kindly remind you of Rule Number Six." At which point the man immediately quieted the entire room by sitting down. A few minutes later, chaos again erupted. This time a woman had stirred things up. Once again, the chairman banged his gavel and reminded her of Rule Number Six. As before, the room instantly settled down. The minister quietly turned to the chairman. "What is Rule Number Six?" he asked.

"Sir," replied the chairman, "Rule Number Six is: Never take yourself, nor anyone else, too seriously."

The minister thought about this tremendously effective rule for a couple of minutes and then leaned over to ask, "What are the other rules?" The chairman chuckled. "There are none," he said.

When it comes to being a lover, who isn't at times constrained by being a father, mother, career holder, or an upstanding member of society? Life is serious business, and it's not easy to find the time to do what it takes to stay creative as a lover. Yet somehow, whenever we do manage to carve out space in our busy lives for sexual play, we are experiencing the light side of our social conditioning.

The truth is, there are many social rules that work well for sexual relationships. As we raise families and participate in community groups, jobs, and social networks, the codes of respect we agree upon allow us to function harmoniously. The trouble is, we forget about our sexual needs, and we get hooked so deeply into our responsibilities that we don't allow ourselves to be lovers too. The question is, regardless of the many roles you play, do you have a leading part as a passionate lover, or do you make an occasional walk-on appearance? Here's how one couple used their social conditioning to their advantage and beat the odds of being bored in the bedroom.

Charlotte and Herb: Breaking Through

I have been married for over fifty years. After we had raised three kids and successfully sent them off into marriages and careers, retirement was a long-awaited breath of fresh air. Finally, I thought, there would be time for hobbies, and even some time for fooling around. Then one day my son-in-law called to tell me he had lost his job, and asked if his kids could stay with us while he and his wife got their life back together. I said yes without hesitation, but then realized the respite I had hoped to enjoy with my husband would need to be put off once again for our grandchildren.

The next day I read on the Internet about a man in his seventies who was making, of all things, high-class porno movies in Japan. If he could make movies, I thought, surely my husband and I could still enjoy sex. I started doing research about senior sex. I even Googled "How to get your groove back after sixty."

It turned out my son-in-law had to delay bringing the kids over to stay. We had an extra two weeks, so I decided we were going to use the time to be lovers in ways we had never done in our whole lives. My husband thought this was a marvelous plan and said he promised to come along for the ride no matter what I came up with.

The next day, I signed up for a weekend sex workshop. We were the oldest couple in the course, but we didn't care one bit. Believe me, being in a room full of people talking about sex was one thing, actually holding and saying lovely things to each other in public, well, it was one of the most exciting things I've ever done. I hadn't felt aroused like that in years! And that was just the talking part . . .

My mother wouldn't have been caught dead doing such a thing, and even my daughter thought we were crazy. But that's the fun part of getting older: people can say what they like; I'm fixing to enjoy whatever years we have left. The energy we stirred up in that sex workshop spilled over into the next week. I was getting breakfast in bed, the yard was raked, and the garbage was taken out before I could say a word. I guess he was hoping to get lucky. It's nice to know that even though we've changed over the years, those warm jazzy feelings are still there. It might take a little longer to get the fire burning, but who cares? Everybody got something good from that workshop. By the time the grandkids rolled up in our driveway, there couldn't have been a happier woman on the planet, or a happier man, for that matter.

Up to this point, social conditioning has mostly been portrayed as a limitation to sexual expression. Conventions that keep us wound up in monotonous routines obviously reinforce the negative aspects of our lover's persona and make it hard to find time for sexual love. Unfortunately we play these parts far too often. But our daily schedules and responsibilities are also marvelous. Whenever we live life on our own terms and break through to enjoy a private liaison of love, we are wearing an empowered face of the Socially Conditioned Lover's Mask. The trick is to treasure moments of sexual tenderness and make them an everyday ritual.

All the lover's masks can be played out in lighthearted ways; and, in fact, even when we venture into the risqué and shadowy sides of sex, if we have the intention to give pleasure and restore harmony, we will gain remarkable insights about who we are. You can use a Lover's Mask in the middle of anything. Try being curious, shy, and then wanton in the kitchen, get seductive at lunchtime, dress like a king or queen for the night. See what it feels like to enjoy the whole pie instead of just a sliver of your Natural Self. Have a few lusty victories, and consider your social conditioning a perfect success.

14

Sustaining the Passion of Intimate Unions

It's no secret that we fare better and learn more by sharing our lives with others. Yet when it comes to improving our intimate unions, we often slide into a laissez-faire attitude, and we leave the utterly central issue of our lives up to chance, hoping things will work themselves out without too much effort. We apply ourselves far more diligently to careers, projects, school, kids, hobbies—just about anything deserves more attention than improving our intimate relationships.

Relationships develop slowly over time through all the incidents, accidents, surprises, and routines, in between the things you never expect to happen and didn't plan for. Once we have found someone endearing enough, and we choose to endure the small and large moments of life together, it's curious how easy it is to drift into a safe harbor and let wave after wave of events dim our awareness and water down passionate feelings. It's comfortable to coast along in daily affairs, becoming more like cohabitating roommates than partners who have it all—financial stability, stimulating communication, and an abundance of sexual intimacy.

Awakening the dynamic potency of an intimate union is not a matter of dissecting everything that happened to you as a child, figuring out why you are shutting down, or picking over past transgressions. Nor is it trying out a few sex tips, buying lingerie, taking another vacation, or finding someone else to have sex with. While these things may or may not temporarily shake things up, Quodoushka shows you different, more compelling ways to share your passion with someone you love.

Keeping the vitality of a relationship alive is a matter of making a commitment to understand how the underlying forces of male and female energy work. When you see what feminine energy is, and what a woman needs to feel alive at the core of her being, and you understand how different a man's needs are, creating a richly potent relationship is not drudgery, it's a pleasure. Rather than slowly and gradually settling for a partnership that drains your life-force energy, you can fulfill your lover's deepest desires for love, sex, and intimate connection by learning to understand what he or she truly needs.

THE ATTRACTION OF DIFFERENCE

While merging money and sex along with sharing our hopes and accomplishments make up the outer features, it's the underlying differences in our instinctual needs that stir the lifeblood of a relationship. Heightening our attraction for each other while sustaining a spiral of deeply loving sexual desire is a matter of going underneath superficial differences to know precisely what our lover truly needs—and then completely giving it. This is what keeps a relationship purring with mystery and lasting affection.

Taoists refer to sexual intercourse as "flowery combat" because the battles between lovers are laced with enticing delicacies of attraction. Will we conquer or surrender? Will we soar freely or graze inside a cozy corral? Great relationships do not boil down differences until intimacy turns into an uninteresting stew of sameness, nor do they flourish in drama after drama. A relationship is not something we enter to win at someone's expense; it's not a competition or a quest for equality. Winning battles and gaining control destroys the desire to intimately engage, and striving for equality, especially in the bedroom, takes away the attraction of difference. Ultimately, we risk this dangerous yet sublime terrain, enduring and enjoying intimate company for one purpose: *to help each other grow.*

Growing in relationship, however, is a confounding and sometimes maddening affair. It's what Nikos Kazantzakis called in *Zorba the Greek* "the full catastrophe." What does a woman want, and what on Earth is feminine energy? What does a man need, and why does he do the things he does? To be sure, what constitutes feminine and masculine qualities is still hotly debated and is not an exact science, but we do not live in scientific debate; we live in the reality that men and women respond, react, and are driven by fundamentally different things. The question is, rather than battling to divide and conquer each other's beauty and power, how do we enhance them? Successful partners instinctively do this—they accentuate, complement, and most of all strengthen each other's masculine and feminine natures. In other words, they use their instinctual differences to become greater by being together.

As we delve into our basic instinctual differences, keep in mind we are not strictly referring to behaviors or societal roles in men and women. We have both masculine and feminine energies in the shields of our luminosity. A woman may exhibit more creative masculine qualities, and a man may exhibit more receptive feminine qualities. Whenever a woman directs her actions with purpose, she is expressing masculine energy, and vice versa. These primal dynamics exist in the same ways between same-sex male and female partners, depending on who is expressing more masculine or feminine energy in the moment.

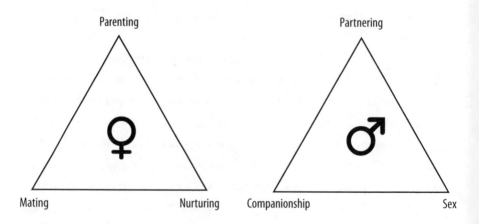

Fig. 14.1. Male Female Basic Instinctual Differences

BASIC INSTINCTUAL DIFFERENCES BETWEEN MEN AND WOMEN

The Feminine Urge to Nurture

Feminine energy seeks to nurture and care for life. It is receptive, like a great bowl that carries and receives whatever is placed inside. Feminine energy resembles the earth's dark, cool soil that holds and nourishes the roots of trees. It's what makes it possible for all of nature to grow, including plants, animals, minerals, and every substance that exists. This is why Quodoushka states, "Everything is born of women."

Because feminine energy is naturally yielding, open, and connected to essentially everything in creation, it is remarkably tuned in to a constant stream of details, feelings, and sensations. Receptivity is anything but passive. In the stillness of waiting, it is mysteriously alive and immeasurably powerful.

The feminine urge to nurture comes with the task of sorting out the complex web of changing impressions that fluctuate within each encounter. It explains why women often feel overwhelmed by the "too-muchness" of what they need to do. It's not that women actually do more than men, it's that women spend tremendous energy wrapping strings of emotional attachment around whatever they care for. A woman's resistance to soften and relax into the vastness of her receptive nature causes her to sag under the weight of her burdens. Taking on too many things at once, she exhausts herself with resentment and peels away the vibrancy of her feminine energy.

Anna's Day

Here's my day. I feel like one of those Shiva sculptures—the ones with about a hundred arms that somehow manage to have a hand in everything. I zip out of bed at 7:00 a.m., feed the kids, make their lunches, get them dressed, and take a quick shower if there's time. Usually I try to talk to my girlfriends about their plans or problems while I clean, fix things around the house, run errands, and shop. Then it's time to get the kids from school, make sure they're all okay, drive them to sports, pick them up, listen to their stories, and make them snacks. By the time my husband gets home and I fix dinner while hearing about his day, I'm exhausted. He works hard too, and we are both pretty tired, so after making sure the homework is done, putting the kids to bed, and cleaning up, I don't have a whole lot of interest in romance, and I don't have much energy for sex either. Falling asleep watching TV is usually the way it goes. By ten o'clock, I'm done. Did I mention I am a part-time flight attendant too? So a few times a month I get to escape for an overnight stay in London or Spain. I'm not complaining, mind you; raising a family is what I want to do.

It's not only women with kids. Add a full-time career to the mix, and the busyness simply expands to fit. I know men who take on child rearing and are surprised by the formidable onslaught of unending tasks that they must cope with. Yet the schedules of modern life are not what create exhaustion; it's how a woman deals with her urge to nurture and how it interferes with her ability to relax that weakens her feminine beauty. When a woman exacerbates her exhaustion with the nagging feelings of not being a good enough partner, mother, or wife, she drains her life-force energy even more. Needless to say, all this takes away her luster in the bedroom.

If a woman does not bring clarity and balance to the way she tries to please others, she will close off her natural feminine abilities and become less and less attractive. In a mature female, nurturing does not mean pleasing everyone at the expense of her own needs. It means choosing to let go of unnecessary entanglements and more carefully selecting when, where, and how to care for others. It also means taking self-care to heart by carving out the time and space in your days to nurture your own intimate sexual needs.

The Masculine Urge for Sex

Masculine energy, on the other hand, resembles the sun's energy. It's warm and penetrating and spreads out like the shining rays of the sun.

Although things may start with receptive feminine energy, nothing goes anywhere without an active masculine spark. This is why Quodoushka states, "Everything is born of feminine energy and is sparked by masculine energy."

Masculine energy is the light of spacious consciousness. When it is focused like a laser with purpose, men can move and finish things with great singular focus. Yet like too much sun on a hot afternoon, it breeds laziness by dispersing itself in frivolous directions. If a man zones out on the couch, switching channels into oblivion, his actions become indecisive, scattered, and incomplete. When masculine energy gets overly fixated, too directed, too excited, or moves too aggressively, it zooms past what's happening and misses the mark entirely. Men may even cross the finish line to achieve the goal, but if they bypass the nuances of pleasure along the way, they are left feeling empty and alone. A strong and mature man extends the focus of his masculine energy with his heart and brings things to fruition with decisive action. In other words, his highest instinct is to serve and protect what matters.

Where a man places his attention and what he does with it is motivated by the current of his innate desire to make sexual connections. The common gripe that "men are only interested in sex" contains a seed of natural truth. Whereas women know themselves through nurturing, men know themselves by making sexual connections. It's not that women don't like sex—they do, but sex and thoughts of sex do not motivate their actions the way they do for men.

Men's focus on sex means that masculine energy is naturally active, outward, and creative. Consider the difference between male and female sexual anatomy. The male member extends outward, and his seeds excitedly move toward the egg, whereas feminine energy primarily floats, lands, and waits to be impregnated. When aroused, masculine energy visibly rises to the occasion. The places where a woman feels pleasure are tucked away inside, spreading inward throughout her entire body. Thus for men, it's not that they actually want to reach out and have sex with everyone they meet. Rather, they instinctively move toward what excites them. What makes them feel most alive? Feminine energy. They know themselves and explore life through the energy they feel at their first chakra—located in their genitals.

Inevitably, though, some male actions and some male sexuality spurts out aimlessly, just as some females in waiting wallow in excessive emotions. The indiscriminate and constant need to feel validated through sex keeps men trapped in unfulfilling connections to the point where the sex they do have is never enough. What clarifies and strengthens a man's energy is the confidence he feels in the core of his sexual being. It's not only the physical act of having sex that brings focus to his wandering heart, and it is untrue that he only needs sex. What he also needs is the acceptance of his creative, sexual nature. This means that when he feels truly welcome, received, and embraced by feminine energy, he can gather his resources, concentrate his actions, and direct his creative ideas with purpose.

When a woman accepts and respects a man's sexual instincts, she doesn't need to fight against his natural inclinations. If she understands that masculine energy needs to move (sometimes in several directions to see what works) and that men are naturally attracted to vibrant sexy energy, she doesn't need to compete with it. A mature woman shines with her inviting, nurturing femininity. As she becomes a magnetic force of sexual warmth, she must also use her intelligence to help him see which of his actions are disconnected from his heart.

She Wants to Mate, He Wants a Companion

This is the universal instinct of hide-and-seek. Think back to when you played this game (which children of all cultures play). Remember the thrill of hiding, searching, and being found? Females like to hide and be found, and males like to hunt and find. A woman is delighted when someone sees that she is special, and she will "mate" with someone who makes her feel like a queen. Men are turned on by the hunt, and they love going out to get game. The male instinct is to search for and then to protect and provide for his companion. The feminine instinct is to create a warm, safe, and secure hearth worthy of protecting.

Although in Australian lingo the word *mate* refers to a buddy, here the feminine instinct of mating means to seek a suitable breeding partner.

When I first heard the Quodoushka teaching that females seek to mate while males want companions, I thought I surely must be a man. I like companions too, and there was no way the drive to produce offspring was the undercurrent to everything I did. Quite frankly, I found the idea of mating archaic and out of tune with my inclinations.

Looking more closely at the meaning, however, I saw that it was true. Take away the idea of mating to produce an actual child, and consider *anything* we create—projects, homes, families, and so forth—as the "children" of our thoughts and actions. With this idea of mating, women seek to bond with whatever they nourish—including the men in their lives. We instinctively attempt to bond with people and situations in order to give birth to something good. Thus, while the feminine instinct to mate includes choosing a potential father, it is also about selecting someone who can help us manifest the "children" of our ideas.

The masculine drive for companionship is different. You could say a companion is a mate with open possibilities. In business, wars, games, and relationships, men create companions and build camaraderie by doing intense, meaningful things with them. They relate and express their love more easily through the things they do together than by the words they say.

Being My Father's Companion

I remember my parents used to call me on the phone while I was in college. After telling my mother the details of everything I was doing, who I was dating, how I liked my roommates, and so on, my father would get on the phone and ask one question: "How's your car?" This went on predictably for years, and I resented him for being so completely unaware of what my life was about. I thought he didn't care.

But then one day it dawned on me what was going on. He was never great with words. I realized that when my father said, "How's your car?" it was his way of saying, "I love you." He wanted me to be safe, and for him, if my car was okay, I was safe. From that moment on, every time he asked about my

car, I joked with him about it. Then I told him how much I really loved him.
It worked, because after a few months of this, he actually said, "I love you" to
my face for the first time. I always knew he loved me because of all the things
he did for me and our family, but hearing him say it, especially when I knew
how hard it was for him, well, it's one of the memories I will see flash before
me when I die. I feel a bit of my father in all the men I care for.

JAMIE

Masculine Freedom versus Feminine Security

In its outward-bound momentum, masculine energy does not like to be hemmed in and needs the freedom to move. It's like a rocket soaring in space that seeks a peaceful place to land once in a while. Freedom from what? Constraints of every kind. It's why men frequently cringe when they are criticized and feel controlled, and yet paradoxically, they also like the attention. If a man strays too far from a rich source of feminine energy, his freedom eventually bores him.

The inward pull of feminine energy is busy making secure nests and seeks places to feel at home. The masculine search for a companion is about finding a partner with whom he wants to share the bounty of the hunt. But what happens if what he returns home with is not desired or sincerely appreciated? And what if a relationship restricts his freedom to keep hunting?

Barbara and George: The Freedom of the Hunt

After two marriages, I have a better idea of what I want in a relationship. I
also know what doesn't work for me anymore. It took me four years to bring
my business to a place where I could afford to move and build the house I
could see myself growing old in. While I was finishing my "castle," I met an
amazing woman named Barbara who I loved being with. She had a home
an hour away from mine and a meaningful career, along with friends and
grandkids of her own. For almost three years, she accompanied me on trips to

various places around the world. I thought we had an excellent situation, and we were very attracted to each other, but then something changed.

For me, the relationship began to fall apart when she started bringing up the idea of living together. Each time I reminded her about the type of living arrangements I wanted, she felt I was avoiding her and not listening to what she wanted. I did hear what she was saying, but I did not want to get married again. I liked having my own home, and I liked going between our two places. The idea of moving into her house, or having her in mine, was out of the question, and I thought I had been clear about that from the beginning. But it was more than this; she started wanting me to change. She became critical of the way I talked to waiters, how I made travel plans, and all sorts of petty things. It reminded me of my marriages, in which I had to compromise about things I didn't even know I was compromising about. Then, one day, I asked her to come with me on a trip to Africa. I had a goal of putting my feet on seven continents by the end of the year, and I had one left to go. When she said, "Why would I want to travel with you just so you can tag another continent?" that was the game-changer. To be fair, she did apologize, but after that, I felt different, and there was no turning back. I guess I have reached a point in my life after seventy years that I want to live a certain way, and I want to be with a woman who supports my dreams.

Her Leap for Independence

Before I turned forty, the main focus of my life was about raising our two sons and taking care of our home. As fifty came in sight, and our sons were nearing graduation, I wanted something more. Up until this time, my husband was the major breadwinner, and while I took part in decisions, in the end Donald decided where the money was spent, where we went on vacations, and what we could afford to do. For years my dream was to have a hair salon. I finally quit my day job, and with my husband's support, I opened my own business with a girlfriend. I can't believe how fabulous it feels to be such a success.

I think it's because the girls at the salon are all really good friends. I never thought much about the way money played a role in our relationship, but now that I am making six figures I am a lot more independent. The downside is that we both work all day, and I sometimes feel like I am just as absent as I used to complain Donald was. What's really difficult is that sex with my husband is pretty much gone, and I want it back. There's no way I want to give up what I am doing, but I don't want to lose my relationship either. One thing I have to say, as I continue to find my way, is that it has meant the world to me that my husband really hung in there for me, even when we were not having much sex.

CAROL

Many women like the rush of economic opportunity and get swept up in the thrills of freedom, new friendships, and making money. In her natural process of evolving, a woman desires to develop her active, creative talents. These are necessary and deeply fulfilling steps in a woman's maturation, but establishing worldly abilities is only a part of her full potential. If a woman stays in this phase of her life and uses her newfound independence to compete with men, her growth will stagnate, and her sexual relationships will flatline. What most women do not realize until they are exhausted, is that at some point during the quest for independence, they have marginalized their need for men and discarded some of their most important feminine graces. For a woman to restore her natural qualities, her challenge is to enjoy the creative intensity of masculine energy by day and be able to slide into bed as a sexy, totally feminine lady at night. Although switching back and forth is not easy, if a woman strays too far from benevolent sources of masculine energy, doing it on her own soon loses its luster.

For her feminine energy to crystallize into captivating beauty, a woman must make a conscious effort to develop the power of her softness. One way to do this is by letting go of the notion that she has to do everything herself. Asking for help, especially from the men in one's life, will allow them show up with more support. In this way, a woman can relax enough to generate power inside her beauty. To avoid becoming too unbalanced, she must not only develop her creativity, she must open herself sexually, too. In other words, she must nourish herself through her sexual expressions and practice being graceful in her creative endeavors. Most importantly, she must find ways to give the love that swells in her being. When she is able to do this, she no longer craves security and no longer needs to prove anything to anyone. As she cares for the warmth and softness of her "home," beauty vibrates through her body, nourishing the wisdom of her heart.

His Inward Dive

I've built several empires from nothing, from restaurants to bars to international charitable foundations. Once I was on vacation in Texas when I noticed there were no great Mexican restaurants in a certain area. In six months I generated the finances, got the real estate, designed the concept, hired the people, and soon had a highly successful enterprise. I know how to make money and make things work. I love doing this, and I have helped many people do it again and again. Why did I leave that restaurant, along with many other thriving businesses and relationships? I don't know. I suppose it was because of a love interest. I am better at starting things than staying with them.

MICHAEL

What happens when a man feels that whatever he is doing is no longer interesting and the things he worked so hard to build collapse? Until he finds what he deeply cares about, his actions flail like weak arrows with nowhere to go. When his masculine energy reserves burn out, he lapses into bouts of indecisiveness and depression and has to hunt for reasons to keep going. If he doesn't go more deeply inward to see what's missing, he will not be able to use his failures and defeats to help him change course. Without finding something he is willing to give his life for, he will spend the rest of his life treading water to stay afloat.

For a man to mature into his full potential he must cast off the tendency to feel rejected and criticized and he must let go of distractions in order to finish things he has started. Then he must harness his creative energy to focus on what is most important. His survival depends on his ability to stand strong even when he feels insecure and alone. If he is to be welcomed warmly by the feminine energy he so desires, he must learn to nurture the territory by being connected to his feelings. He must open to new expressions of his sexuality by becoming more sensitive and caring as a lover. When he is steadfast in his commitments, he develops the ability to withstand the seemingly endless tests that life (and especially women) invariably throw his way. As he takes a stand to live on his own terms with a receptive heart, he will find that his instincts to defend, protect, and serve are truly needed. He no longer needs to break free from constraints or possess things to prove his worth. Everything he does with compassion and passion are the gifts of his masculine essence.

THE WHEEL OF RELATIONSHIP FOCUS

The expression of masculine and feminine energies evolves and changes as we grow through relationships. We gain energy from the differences in our instinctual natures by shifting from Self-Focus into Relationship Focus. Strengthening our own internal masculine and feminine abilities propels us into Merging and Cohesion Focus, until we enter the dynamic harmony of what is called Warrior Focus.

To mature as a man means to develop and embrace feminine energy, both your own and your partner's. The key is to do things that increase your sensitivity and that help you become more open and receptive. What kinds of things? Martial arts, meditation, dancing, gardening, caring for children, music—anything that teaches you how to navigate through complex, subtle feelings.

To mature as a woman means to embrace masculine energy—your own and your partner's. This has little do with sexual preferences. You can receive masculine energy and form intimate alliances with any man in

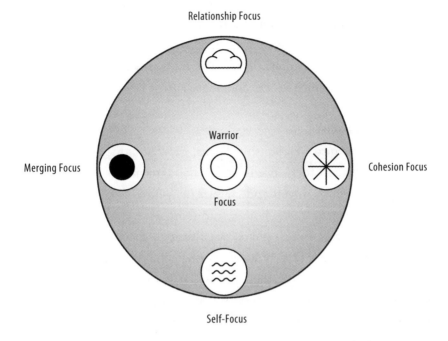

Relationship Focus

Merging Focus

Warrior

Focus

Cohesion Focus

Self-Focus

Fig. 14.2. The Wheel of Relationship Focus

your life, including brothers, friends, or lovers. To enhance your feminine potency, you must develop the ability to clarify your emotions, select your focus, and then move with decisive actions. Knowing how to cultivate our own inner masculine and feminine energies not only increases attraction within intimate relationships—it changes the way we relate to all men and women.

Self-Focused Relationships

Immature men and women pit their needs and desires against each other in Self-Focused, needy relationships that consist of two people lost in their own worlds gathering self-indulgent resentments. Both partners are unwilling and unable to admit their real desires and are entirely focused on getting their own needs met. Giving is mostly about "What's in this for me?" Self-Focused relationships are marked by denial, secrecy, lying, betrayal, laziness, jealousy, repulsion, and a sense of trying to get even. When we are trapped inside Self-Focused relationships, we sabotage intimacy because we feel we don't deserve it. This is why sex is mostly a disappointing battle in which, in the end, more energy is lost than gained.

Relationship Focus

When we enter into Relationship Focus, we communicate with greater awareness of each other's needs and make agreements for more equal exchanges. For both singles and couples, it is often a highly productive period for building careers, homes, and families, and also for exploring new sexual interests. In this phase, by cultivating their opposite qualities, both partners mature as they break through the restraints of their own gender. As women actualize their creative talents and men delve into their sensations, relationships are about learning to give and receive in more mutually satisfying ways. Sex is more appealing, pleasurable, and caring.

It sounds wonderful, yet Relationship Focus is typically the most challenging phase in any relationship. While we are trying to be less selfish and we get better at expressing ourselves, we are still vying for equality of status. Everything, it seems, has to be equal; a career should be as important as housework, money should be equally divided, and there should be equal satisfaction when it comes to sex.

During this period, which can last for years, expressing our sexual needs is rarely a smooth process. Negotiations often turn into tedious, endless debates, constant bickering or long bouts of withdrawal. It's is a confusing time, because just as we are trying so hard to articulate what we need and we are trying to understand each other better, the very qualities we are cultivating in order to grow weaken our sexual attraction. As men seek to become more sensitive and caring, they become less focused and more indecisive. As women develop their assertiveness and independence, they become more powerful and less sexually available.

In Neuro-Linguistic Programming (NLP), one of the methods for creating rapport is to become like your opponents. You mime their gestures and mimic the cadence of their voice so completely that you understand their motivations to the point you can actually feel the way they do. In intimate relations, however, becoming too much like the other takes away the very things we are most attracted to.

This is the phase inside Relationship Focus when many intelligent men and women with accomplished careers or secure families reach a period of stasis. It's the place in a relationship where it feels like something is seriously missing. Sexual desire and frequency decreases, and it feels as if growth has stopped. Although we have developed better communication skills, our basic instinctual needs are starving for expression. We crave more intimate sexual and intellectual stimulation. Women who are in Relationship Focus typically say they want more sensitive men, or may complain that there are "no good men out there." Even if they have a partner, they start desiring stronger expressions of masculine energy. And while men in Relationship Focus often say they like powerful women, they also begin to want more available, carefree, and easygoing feminine energy. There's no stopping this mutual quest to mature, however. When men hunker down to nest, make commitments, and accept responsibilities, they become more feminine; and when women become interested in independence, success, and freedom, they become more masculine. Many relationships idle in this position, and it is at this juncture that partners frequently spiral into divorces or drift into separate universes. Whether partners stay together or not, each has the opportunity to shift his or her focus and rise to a different way of relating.

Merging into Cohesion Focus

What can we do when growth seems to be at a standstill and daily irritations make it impossible to connect? As when we watch a plant, we can't always see when we are growing, but we do know when we feel squelched inside a relationship. Recurring fights and escalating conflicts are signs that your instinctual needs are not being met and that you are stuck moving back and forth between Self-Focus and Relationship Focus.

Moving from Merging Focus into Cohesion Focus is not a fairy tale of becoming one with the other or landing serenely in a constant state of happiness with someone you love. It does not mean the end of differences.

In fact, as you enter Merging Focus, male-female instinctual differences are even more distinct. Merging Focus is like navigating through a maze that requires both partners to develop more mature expressions of their masculine and feminine essences. Gradually, as women embrace the grace and power of their femininity and men persevere with compassion, sex becomes far more pleasurable and fulfilling.

Moving Through the Maze:
Dissolving Conflict into Attraction

In the initial stages of Merging Focus, you must admit your hidden fears and go right into the places that scare you the most. If you are afraid of losing control, go into that, talk about it. If you are afraid of being left alone or betrayed, or you are furious about being lied to, admit your hidden fears. If you are jealous or bored, or you are worried about sexual performance, talk about these things. Underneath these issues is always the fear of loss. To transcend it, you need to name what you are afraid of losing. When we stay in Relationship Focus, we go back and forth trying to change what we don't like about each other. Most of the time we battle behind a smokescreen of unresolved points of contention and avoid asking for what we truly need and desire. This is what causes us to separate in anguish and bitter disappointment.

Merging into Cohesion Focus takes you toward what you can't stand about your partner. Rather than recoiling, or trying to get the other to change, you start to merge with whatever annoys you. Let's say it's how he or she always yells. Even if you have heard it a thousand times, listen to it. Really hear it. Or let's say it's how he or she withdraws and sulks. Instead of defending your position, or trying to change your partner, become deliberately receptive and open. In Relationship Focus, you talk about what irritates you, try to take responsibility for what's yours, and make agreements not to do it again. Usually, although intentions are good, agreements don't last. When you are moving into Cohesion Focus, you start to listen to and feel what the other feels. You feel the pain they feel when they withdraw. You feel your lover's stress and try to see what he or she actually needs. If you can deliberately move closer to what you find unattractive, you will automatically step outside of your own Self-Focus.

Warrior Focus

When you face your worst fears and are no longer run by a sense of loss, you begin to enter Cohesion Focus and gain glimpses of Warrior Focus. The practice is to shift your awareness onto the other and give what you are most afraid of losing. If you are afraid of being left, be more intimate. If you need sexual release, be more passionate in what you do. If you crave security, give someone the safety of your friendship by being a better friend. If you need space, find a way to give it. You may not get exactly what you want in the way you want it when you want it. Relationships rarely work so evenly. Within Cohesion Focus you will, however, find yourself drawn to share what you have rather than fighting for what you don't. You needn't wait to have a beloved to enter Cohesion Focus and sometimes you may even separate in a loving manner. While this seems like a contradiction, Cohesion Focus does not necessarily mean you will always remain with your partner. The practice is to cherish moments of intimacy by giving tenderly what you most desire, and giving away what you are most attached to.

Finally, healing conflicts and restoring the potency of your relations within Warrior Focus means to feel your partner's desires more keenly than your own. Seek to see, understand, and know what her needs are and strive to give them. See what his needs are and find a way to give without wanting anything back. Striving to feel and give what the other needs, even if it means sacrificing something you want for yourself, becomes far more attractive than your own gratification. This is particularly true when it comes to sex, where surrendering to the bliss of pleasure brings you face to face with every vulnerability, insecurity, and fear you've ever known. Warrior Focus takes us into the abyss of the unknown and keeps us continually experiencing new edges of awareness.

The Final Instinctual Difference: Parenting and Partnering

As we move from Self-Focus toward Cohesion Focus and Warrior Focus, division between masculine and feminine energies fuses into mutual desire for the other to stand fully in their greatness. The feminine instinct to parent is the compassionate desire to turn the men she knows into "gods," and the masculine instinct is to cherish and protect life itself by supporting the women in his life to become "goddesses."

A woman brings forth the most expansive qualities from the men in her life not by excusing careless actions or by cutting them down. A mature woman inspires something better. She treats men with dignity, and she is honored in return. A woman who has cultivated her feminine energy with mastery neither craves nor demands security for herself; she is secure, even in the face of suffering heartbreaking devastation and loss. Her task is to test and challenge masculine energy (including her own) in such a way that the most life-affirming choices, decisions, and solutions survive. As she learns to clarify her emotions, she can suggest options rather than make demands. Then she must give the men in her life the space to figure things out on their own. In this way, she becomes confident and magnetic, and she welcomes the vulnerability of opening herself to masculine energy whenever she wants to.

In a mature male, every woman in a sense becomes his partner, a goddess whom he desires to protect and provide for. While providing for others, however, he must also learn to care for himself. He does this by gaining command over his own childish emotions and by encouraging the women in his life to express their individuality and freedom. As he actualizes his dreams, he becomes more self-assured and thus inspires the women in his life to become more relaxed in expressing their femininity.

His energy is not distracted, chasing to possess whatever attracts him in the moment. Sex is no longer a need for release, or a brief respite; it becomes the concentration of his pure desire to pour his energy into life. The games of hunting to conquer no longer interest him, not because he has given up, but because the real hunt is for his courage to choose when, where, and how he can offer his gifts fully in service to others. Having or not having sex does not dominate his thoughts. By developing discernment, he acquires the foresight to see the consequences of his actions. He ages with maturity by learning to generously respect and honor the beauty of feminine energy. Though his battles with inner and outer demons may never end, his dignity prevails.

When the questions "What do we want?" "What do we need?" and "What makes us different?" are answered—not with certain conclusions, but by an even greater desire to understand ourselves and each other—sexual intimacy becomes a source of unending discovery. Whenever we rise from defeat and let go of something we thought we couldn't survive without, we take a step up on the ladder of evolution. The secret is to know there is no final destination and to realize how we truly need each other to learn and grow. As we evolve together in this way, sex is sacred not because it's fantastic every time, because you know a certain technique, or because you finally have a great partner; it's because you have changed.

15

CREATING A SACRED
SEXUAL CEREMONY

APPROACHING SEX IN A MORE SACRED WAY

We've all heard that the best way to sustain a great relationship is to make sure sex is good. Supposedly, somewhere, behind closed doors, fortunate couples are doing it. Less commonly known is what they actually do to achieve a more sexually fulfilling relationship. One of the easiest and most effective ways to bring your sexuality to a higher level is to create an inspiring intention together.

Lovemaking can be a quick grasp for a temporary surge of pleasure, or, if you take the time to share more carefully considered intentions, you can make love in a way that brings your hearts, bodies, minds, and spirits into alignment. Co-creating an intent before, during, and after lovemaking brings meaning and passion to your sexual unions. Feelings of sweetness and overflowing gratitude will naturally pass between you. Each and every embrace becomes food for your soul's delight. Establishing clear intentions through ceremony harnesses and directs the forces of your sexual energy for a greater purpose. You become a generous, loving cell within the body of Great Spirit by helping your partner embody his or her full potential with balanced masculine and feminine energy.

Sharing the following gains or gifts can turn any encounter into a healing expression of your sexual love. Each statement is about the gifts you gain by giving and receiving inspiring thoughts of beauty. Read them before making love and talk about them afterward to bask in the warmth of connected conversation. Talk about the gifts that touch you most and see how the quality of your lovemaking changes.

THE WHEEL OF BEAUTY

East

By choosing to make love with passion and lust, we gain the gift of Creative Originality.

West

By totally getting into the pure feelings of intimate sex, we gain the gifts of Prowess and Strength.

South

By letting go of things from the past, and giving to one another with tenderness, we gain the gift of Fluid, Sensuous Intimacy.

North

By sharing empowering beliefs about sex and bringing humor into our love life, we gain the gift of Flexible Clarity.

Southwest

By being open to discovering new things we like, and coming together as if for the first time, we gain the gift of being Inquisitive Explorers.

Southeast

By accepting ourselves, being vulnerable, and sharing what we find beautiful about each other, we gain the gift of Individuality.

Northwest

By changing patterns that are not working for us and doing what we love, we gain the gift of Autonomy.

Northeast

By relaxing and focusing on being more spontaneous, we gain the gift of Free Will.

Center

By being completely honest about our needs and desires, and having sex more often, we gain the gifts of Liberty and Freedom.

CREATING YOUR SEXUAL CEREMONY

This ceremony is a way of making your union a special occasion. To enhance your lovemaking, you can bring the elements of creation into your home to create an altar of love. Placing the elements of water, earth, wind and fire together in this way brings us back to the essence of what created us. Taking the time to select and place the following elements into your own wheel is a way of showing how much you care for each other. By doing this together, you are co-creating an intention to share a joyful celebration of sexual intimacy.

◎ Creating a Simple Love Altar

You can create this altar on a small table near where you will make love.

South

Water and Emotions

Find a small, lovely bowl and fill it with water. You can also put a flower into the bowl. Place it on a table in the South position, or on a blanket especially chosen for your sexual ceremony. The water represents giving with tenderness.

North

Wind and Mind

Place a piece of incense in an incense holder in the North. Wait to light it until just before lovemaking. This represents your mind and the wind. It will assist you in brushing away distractions and calming your mind so you can focus totally on giving and receiving pleasure. It will also help you gain knowledge about what your lover needs most in the moment. The incense represents receiving with care.

West

Earth and Body

Find another small bowl and fill it with earth. Place it in the West of your wheel. It will help get you into your body and allow you to fully enjoy the sensations of touch. Earth represents the physical body and will remind you to trust your intuitions to find the kinds of touch your lover most desires. This is the place of holding and transforming with intimacy.

East

Fire and Spirit

In the East of your altar, place a candle. Wait to light it just before you are ready to make love. Fire represents the expansiveness of your being. It shows us the beauty of passion. The ceremony celebrates the spirit of your union, the Quodoushka energy that joins to create more than the sum of individual parts. Thus, no mater how you come together, you can grow and learn by sharing the most precious energy in the world, your sexual energy. The candle reminds you to determine your desires with passion and lust.

Center

Soul and Void

In the center of your altar, put something special that carries a particular meaning to you both. It could be a picture, or even a dream you wish to manifest. You can also place a note in the center where you have written the way you feel about each other. The void is the both the emptiness and fullness from which everything comes into existence and through which everything returns. Enjoy the moments of connection and inspire each other to share natural affection and love. This is the place where you catalyze your sexuality with heart-to-heart communication.

Once you have read the Wheel of Beauty and have arranged your altar, make love in any way you like. Note: Remember Rule Number Six: Don't take yourself, or anything else, too seriously. Have fun, be spontaneous, and enjoy.

To complete your ceremony there are a few final steps. The first is to offer a small gift from your heart to your partner while thanking him or her for sharing this special time with you. The second is to cleanse the space with as much care as you created it. With thoughts or words of gratitude, give the water to a plant, return the earth to the ground, blow out the candle, and clear away the incense. Finally, if you have written down a dream you wish to manifest or if you have a photograph or a token used in your ceremony, there are several things you can do to bring closure in a good way. You can burn the item, put it in a special place, or let it go by releasing it into the wind.

Afterword

Who we truly are is far greater than who we wish to be.

THUNDER STRIKES

In many ways, this statement captures the essence of what Quodoushka is all about. For once we gain a sense of how we can change our lives by improving our attitude and approach to sex, it leaves us in appropriate wonder about who we truly are. There is so much more to our intimate lives than wanting to have better sex. Yet, feeling the urgency of intimacy and knowing how disconnected we feel when we don't have it is the first step toward liberation. It is my sincere hope that through reading this book, many will be inspired to learn through pleasure and find a path with heart where sex is considered natural, healthy, and good.

One of the difficulties I have in presenting this material is the realization that written words can only point to the kind of healing and transformation that happen when Quodoushka is personally shared between teachers and students. To gain the full impact of these practices, I hope that many will find the guidance they need to become more balanced human beings. (A list of resources is located in the back of this book.) For as we experience Quodoushka to understand the depth of our personal vulnerabilities and collective conflicts surrounding sex, we begin to realize that each of us deserves pleasure and that repressing our Natural Self only diminishes our experience of life.

As we share these teachings with our families, friends, and lovers, they can serve as a kind of rite of passage into a world of greater Hope, Happiness, Humor, Health, and Harmony. Yet, if we are to live in such a world, and grow as a mature, tolerant, and wise society, how can we continue to neglect teaching our children what they need to know about their sexuality? We can no longer afford to leave one of the most important aspects of our lives to chance. We need to become whole again by embracing our sexuality with greater knowledge, compassion, responsibility, and freedom. This is what it means to heal ourselves first, and in this way, give to the next seven generations in beauty.

Resources

AUTHORIZED QUODOUSHKA TEACHERS

John Ardagh: www.quodoushka.com, thunderwolf@sympatico.ca.

Barbara Brachi: www.icss.org, icss@tcn.ca.

Amara Charles: www.amaracharles.com, amara@amaracharles.com.

Rose Fink: www.quodoushka.co.uk, fynkin@aol.com.

Batty Gold: www.quodoushka.co.uk, battygold@aol.com.

Janneke Koole: www.quodoushka.com, beyondwords@me.com.

Karen Krauss: www.quodoushka.com, swmedicine@aol.com.

Asa Kullberg: www.quodoushka.com, littlesword@swipnet.se.

Mary Minor: www.quodoushka.com, medicinedirector@dtmms.org.

Ina Mlekush: www.spiritualsexuality.com, Ina@SpiritualSexuality.com.

Mukee Okan: www.spiritfireproductions.com, mukee@spiritfireproductions.
   com.

Kristin Viken: www.quodoushka.com, kristin@shamanicdearmoring.com.

QUODOUSHKA WORKSHOPS OF THE DEER TRIBE METIS MEDICINE SOCIETY (DTMMS) AND AFFILIATES

Australia: www.ozsacredsexuality.com. (011-64-1300-38-2877)

Canada: www.icss.org. (416-603-4912)

Europe: www.dtmms-europe.com. (011-49-338-469-0574)

United States: www.dtmms.org. and www.quodoushka.com. (480-443-3851)

ᴎ⊙ᴛᴇꜱ

INTRODUCTION. THE MEDICINE OF SEX—
LEARNING THROUGH PLEASURE

1. Susy Buchanan, "Sacred Orgasm," *Phoenix New Times,* June 13, 2002.

CHAPTER 1. THE LEGACY OF QUODOUSHKA

1. Hyemeyhosts Storm, *Lightning Bolt* (New York: Random House, 1994), 290–348.
2. Ibid.

CHAPTER 6. A NATURAL LANGUAGE FOR SEX

1. Paul Joannides, *Guide to Getting It On* (Waldport, Ore.: Goofy Foot Press, 2009), 86–87.
2. Ibid., 188–89.
3. Ibid., 94–99.
4. Ibid., 188–89.

CHAPTER 8. FEMALE GENITAL ANATOMY TYPES

1. Ted Andrews, *Animal-Speak: The Spiritual and Magical Powers of Creatures Great and Small* (St. Paul, Minn.: Llewellen, 1903), 258, 259.

2. Andrews, *Animal-Speak,* 250–252.

3. Ibid., 271–272.

4. Ibid., 262–264.

CHAPTER 9. MALE GENITAL ANATOMY TYPES

1. Paul Joannides, *Guide to Getting It On* (Waldport, Ore.: Goofy Foot Press, 2009), 41–50.

2. Ted Andrews, *Animal-Speak: The Spiritual and Magical Powers of Creatures Great and Small* (St. Paul, Minn.: Llewellen, 1903), 251.

3. Jan Orsi, Thunder Strikes, *Song of the Deer: The Great SunDance Journey of the Soul* (Malibu, Calif.: Jaguar Books, Inc., 1999), 174, 175.

4. Andrews, *Animal-Speak,* 270.

5. Ibid., 307, 308.

CHAPTER 12. SEXUAL HEALING PRACTICES

1. www.benunderwood.com/index.html.

2. www.benunderwood.com/aboutme.html.

3. Thunder Strikes with John Kent, *Shamanic De-armoring Manual* (Phoenix, Ariz.: The Deer Tribe Metis Medicine Society [DTMMS] 2007), 48, 49, 69.

Index

Page numbers in *italics* refer to illustrations.

BOOKS OF RELATED INTEREST

The Complete Illustrated Kama Sutra
Edited by Lance Dane

Healing Love through the Tao
Cultivating Female Sexual Energy
Mantak Chia

Lingam Massage
Awakening Male Sexual Energy
Michaela Riedl and Jürgen Becker

Yoni Massage
Awakening Female Sexual Energy
Michaela Riedl

The Sexual Herbal
Prescriptions for Enhancing Love and Passion
Brigitte Mars, A.H.G.

Slow Sex
The Path to Fulfilling and Sustainable Sexuality
Diana Richardson

Tantric Sex for Men
Making Love a Meditation
Diana Richardson and Michael Richardson

Tantric Orgasm for Women
Diana Richardson

INNER TRADITIONS • BEAR & COMPANY
P.O. Box 388
Rochester, VT 05767
1-800-246-8648
www.InnerTraditions.com

Or contact your local bookseller